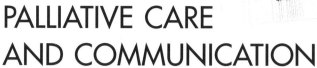

PALLIATIVE CARE
AND COMMUNICATION

FACING DEATH

Series editor: David Clark, Professor of Medical Sociology, University of Sheffield

The subject of death in late modern culture has become a rich field of theoretical, clinical and policy interest. Widely regarded as a taboo until recent times, death now engages a growing interest among social scientists, practitioners and those responsible for the organization and delivery of human services. Indeed, how we die has become a powerful commentary on how we live and the specialized care of dying people holds an important place within modern health and social care.

This series captures such developments. Among the contributors are leading experts in death studies, from sociology, anthropology, social psychology, ethics, nursing, medicine and pastoral care. A particular feature of the series is its attention to the developing field of palliative care, viewed from the perspectives of practitioners, planners and policy analysts; here several authors adopt a multi-disciplinary approach, drawing on recent research, policy and organizational commentary, and reviews of evidence-based practice. Written in a clear, accessible style, the entire series will be essential reading for students of death, dying and bereavement and for anyone with an involvement in palliative care research, service delivery or policy making.

PALLIATIVE CARE AND COMMUNICATION

Experiences in the clinic

ANNE-MEI THE

OPEN UNIVERSITY PRESS
Buckingham · Philadelphia

Open University Press
Celtic Court
22 Ballmoor
Buckingham
MK18 1XW

email: enquiries@openup.co.uk
world wide web: www.openup.co.uk

and
325 Chestnut Street
Philadelphia, PA 19106, USA

First Published 2002

This edition was originally published as: Anne-Mei The (1999) *Palliatieve behandeling en communicatie: een onderzoek naar het optimisme op herstel van longkankerpatienten.* Houten: Bohn Stafleu Van Laghum.
The English edition was translated from the Dutch by Robert Pool.

A catalogue record of this book is available from the British Library

ISBN 0 335 21205 0 (pb)   0 335 21206 9 (hb)

Library of Congress Cataloging-in-Publication Data
The, Anne-Mei.
    [Palliatieve behandeling en communicatie. English]
    Palliative care and communication: experiences in the clinic/Anne-Mei The.
        p. cm – (Facing death)
    Includes bibliographical references and index.
    ISBN 0–335–21206–9 – ISBN 0–335–21205–0 (pbk.)
    1. Lungs–Cancer–Netherlands. 2. Medical personnel and patient–Netherlands. 3. Terminal care–Netherlands. 4. Lungs—Cancer—Palliative treatment—Netherlands. 5. Cancer–Psychological aspects. I. Title.
    II. Series.

RC280.L8 T48 2002
616.99′42406′09492—dc21   2001059113

Typeset by Graphicraft Limited, Hong Kong
Printed in Great Britain by Biddles Limited, Guildford and Kings Lynn

Contents

Series editor's preface

It is a particular pleasure to introduce this work from Anne-Mei The, which marks one dozen volumes in the Facing Death series since we began in 1997. Her book wonderfully complements two other ethnographic studies that we have already published. It can be read alongside a detailed analysis of the management of death in the intensive care unit (Seymour 2001) and it is also a fascinating counterpoint to an enquiry into the 'calendars of treatment' experienced by cancer patients as they pick their way through an array of services and settings (Costain Schou and Hewison 1999). *Palliative Care and Communication: Experiences in the Clinic* thereby adds to our growing understanding of end of life issues as seen from the multiple perspectives of those who receive care and those who give it. Indeed it invites us to reappraise radically many of our previous notions of care 'delivery'.

Anne-Mei The is a cultural anthropologist of consummate skill. She takes us inside a world of paradoxes and tensions where those with lung cancer seek to make sense of their experience of a life threatening illness. In doing this she uncovers a remarkable paradox: when confronted with a disease that is almost invariably and often swiftly fatal, patients nevertheless maintain a remarkable sense of optimism about the future. Why this should be, how it is viewed by others, and the consequences that ensue, are the core issues which this book tackles. Anne-Mei The does this by accompanying 30 patients from the time they 'learn' of their fatal prognosis, until death. She attends meetings and consultations, maintains contact with patients in the clinic, on the ward and at home, indeed is present as patients receive active treatment. Her abilities in listening and observing in these varied settings are matched by the eloquence with which she writes. Never cloying, patronizing or melodramatic, she succeeds admirably in capturing atmosphere, context, background 'noise' and complexity. Moreover, she is a rare example of a researcher who is prepared to present her findings in a narrative which reflects the research process itself and the insights gained along the way – a technique long ago advocated by the 'Chicago school' of sociology, but not often seen in action. The result is a hugely engaging and compassionate journey of discovery for the reader, both through the world of lung cancer care and also into the researcher's own actions and thought processes – especially as her work shifts over time from what she describes as an 'information perspective' to that of a 'care perspective'.

Anne-Mei The has chosen the single entity of lung cancer to study and that is welcome in providing a level of detail about the specifics of this particular disease. She has also picked a cancer that has attracted less research interest than some others. Her fieldwork was carried out in the Netherlands, but the disease she describes and the experiences of those who encounter it are undoubtedly generalizable to many other settings and contexts. At the same time there are valuable insights into the way in which one health care system and culture deals with a disease that is widespread and increasing throughout the world. I am delighted to introduce *Palliative Care and Communication* to the Facing Death series and have no hesitation in commending this excellent book to our growing readership.

David Clark

References

Costain Schou, K. and Hewison, J. (1999) *Experiencing Cancer: Quality of Life in Treatment*. Buckingham: Open University Press.

Seymour, J.E. (2001) *Critical Moments: Death and Dying in Intensive Care*. Buckingham: Open University Press.

Acknowledgements

Research and writing are not individual activities. Many people were involved in the conception of this book. Some of them have influenced my work to such an extent that I want to thank them personally: the patients and their relatives who admitted me to such an emotional and dramatic period in their lives; the doctors and nurses who had the courage to allow me to observe them. They have given me more wisdom about being ill and dying and all its related complexities than I will ever be able to glean from books. Gerard Koëter guided me through the intricacies of practice. Without his support and our many conversations both my career in and my thinking about health care would have been completely different. Tony Hak taught me much about qualitative research and medical sociology. His clear vision was not only invaluable in analysing my results but also inspiring. Robert Pool provided important comments on the Dutch edition of this book. He translated it into English and once again suggested useful improvements. The series editor, David Clark, and Jacinta Evans and Maureen Cox of Open University Press not only made the English edition of the book possible, they did so in a very efficient and pleasant manner. Finally I would also like to mention Marleen Bakker, Suzanne Bogman, Harry Groen, Tjeerd Tijmstra, The Tjwan Hauw, Marjan Verkerk, Ruurd Veldhuis, Gerrit van der Wal and Onno Zeylstra. They know why.

The research on which this book is based was financed by the Dutch Cancer Society and the SKWOSZ Foundation (Slotervaart ziekenhuis). NWO (the Netherlands Organisation for Scientific Research) financed the English translation.

Introduction

Mr van der Ploeg

The man sitting next to me in the waiting room leans over, 'It's unbeliev-able,' he says. 'That cancer has disappeared completely: Dr Liem says I'm cured'. I look at him questioningly. 'Is he serious?' I wonder. Mr van der Ploeg returns my gaze calmly and nods. His hand searches for that of his wife, while she fiddles with her handkerchief. 'We're so happy,' she says, through the tears. I look at them in disbelief: they really seem to think that he has been cured. What is going on?

It was January 1993, and for the past six months I had been in the Ruysdael Clinic studying how euthanasia and other related end-of-life deci-sions develop (The 1996, 1997a, 1998). I was initially based on the wards, carrying out participant observation, mainly among the nurses. When euthanasia did occur on the wards, the preparatory discussions between doctor and patient had often already taken place during consultations in the outpatient clinic, so hoping to experience some of these discussions first-hand, I had extended my activities to the outpatient clinic.

Sitting there in the waiting room next to Mr and Mrs van der Ploeg, I recalled the words of the head of the outpatient clinic for lung diseases, 'Do you realize that if you walk into this clinic in 18 months' time, most of the patients you see now will be dead?' he asked. Mr van der Ploeg's words exercised me the rest of the morning. Had I misunderstood the prognosis? I consulted the handbook 'Longziekten' (Lung Diseases) (Postmus 1993): 'Untreated, all lung carcinomas are fatal,' I read. 'In the case of small-cell anaplastic carcinoma, the median survival after diagnosis is three months.' I scan down the page. 'The rate of growth of small-cell lung carcinoma is phenomenal, the tumour may double in size every 30 days. In almost all cases metastases are already present at first diagnosis.' Mr van der Ploeg had liver metastases. 'Small-cell lung carcinoma is very responsive to chemo-therapy . . . often the disease-free interval can be extended. . . . However, the long-term results are disappointing. . . . Generally the prognosis remains poor. Most patients who cannot be operated on die within two years. . . .' Nine months previously Mr van der Ploeg was diagnosed as having meta-stasized small-cell lung carcinoma. He claimed to be cured; the book said he could not have much time left.

I closed the book and walked to the door of the waiting room. A doctor emerged from a consulting room and beckoned a patient, who followed him inside. Above the closed door a light went on. Patients sat on artist-ically arranged designer chairs against a backdrop of colourful murals by young artists. Birds sang high up in the branches of indoor palm trees. Ubiquitous signs of modernity. No expense had been spared in the effort to banish any suggestion of disease, suffering and death from the Ruysdael Clinic and make it pleasant for patients. At the far end I saw Mr van der Ploeg making a new appointment at the reception desk: a checked cap covered his bald head, his jacket was loose – he had lost a lot of weight during the months of chemotherapy. 'It's unbelievable, Dr Liem says I'm cured,' reverberated through my head.

I remembered the lectures on health-care law that I had attended in preparation for this study. The law prohibits a care provider from initiating or continuing treatment without the informed consent of the patient. In 1995 this was subsumed under a new law (WGBO, *Wet op de Genees-kundige Behandelings Overeenkomst*). This law, like the renovation of the hospital itself, was an expression of the transition of the health-care sector to the modern age. The law was intended to make the relationship between doctor and patient more open, egalitarian and cooperative (Leenen 1995: i), to improve communication and to improve the patient's legal position (Legemaate 1995: xi). The right to information was meant to enable the patient to evaluate his or her own situation and form a balanced judgement about treatment and lifestyle. The doctor's obligation to provide informa-tion included counselling about prognosis (Roscam Abbing 1995: 25). If Mr van der Ploeg really believed that his treatment was curative rather than palliative, and that he was indeed cured, where did that leave informed consent?

Research question, methods and presentation

On that January morning in 1993 the idea was born for the study on which this book is based. In the outpatient clinic I had not found what I had expected: patients did not appear to be exercised by their approaching demise. On the contrary, patients and their relatives, like Mr and Mrs van der Ploeg, seemed optimistic about recovery and made plans for the future. When I mentioned this 'unjustified optimism' to doctors and nurses, they readily agreed that it was a problem, but I never received a satisfactory explanation. Doctors simply said, 'That's how patients are'. Nurses blamed inadequate counselling by the doctors, but admitted that they were never actually present when this occurred. During counselling sessions that I attended, I did hear doctors inform patients that their illness was incurable. So why were they unjustifiably optimistic? What was it in the communication between doctors, patients and nurses that caused patients to be oblivious to what was obvious to their care providers?

In order to understand what was happening I tried to put myself in the position of each of the various protagonists and see their point of view. In initial, exploratory discussions I was struck by the differences in perspective between doctors and nurses, and it seemed a good idea to study the views of doctors and nurses who were involved with the same patient and the same illness episode. Using the ethnographic method, I followed 30 patients from the moment they first received the news that they were incurably ill until their death. In this way I automatically came into contact with all the care providers who were involved in a particular patient's care. Between 1993 and 1997 I studied two cycles of 15 patients each. I attended consultations and staff discussions, participated in ward rounds, was present during treatment and chemotherapy, and sat with relatives in waiting rooms. I also maintained contact with patients when they were outside the hospital, either by phoning or visiting them at home.

Anyone could potentially find themselves in the position of the incurably ill patients in this study; hence, the subject of this book is also of relevance to those outside the medical profession. With this in mind it has been written in an accessible, narrative style. I tell the 'whole story': by presenting the full context, atmosphere, chaos, background noise and complexity, I hope to make the events understandable to the layperson, familiar to the insider and convincing for all. By writing from within, extensively and with empathy, about the daily routine in the Lung Department, by describing in detail what I saw and experienced, I hope to engender in the reader a detailed picture and an understanding of local rationality.

Rather than presenting results based on the knowledge and understanding that I gained retrospectively, after I had collected and analysed all the data, I follow my own journey of discovery during the study. I have chosen this format because it is the logical trajectory that a layperson would follow in practice. But there is also a methodological reason. An important aspect of qualitative research is that the researcher 'learns' during the research process. As a result he adjusts his approach and his research questions as he goes along, rather than slavishly following a predetermined protocol. In my case, the learning process was characterized by a change of perspective. I started from what I call an *information perspective*, looking predominantly at what people said and how they said it. As the study progressed, I began develop more of an eye for the influence of the patient on the process of communication, and for the interaction between care providers and patient. The information perspective became less useful for analysing what was going on and I gradually changed to what I call a *care perspective*.

The book

The complete illness trajectories of Mr Dekker and Mr Wiersema form the backbone of the book, and these are supplemented with details from the trajectories and experiences of other patients. Mr Dekker and Mr Wiersema are fictional, but their personalities and illness trajectories are based on those of real people. In order to guarantee confidentiality I have changed the names, characteristics and illness trajectories of patients and woven fictional characters and events from threads taken from different real cases and events. The descriptions are annotated, and I have typologically distinguished descriptive text from discussion, so that readers who simply want to follow the narrative can easily do so, and those who would like some deeper reflection can also find their way.

The book is divided into five parts. The first four parts each present a phase of the illness trajectory. Part I describes the first phase, in which the doctor informs the patient of the diagnosis, and in which first-line chemotherapy is central. Chapter 1 presents three variations on the 'bad news interview' in which the patient is told that he or she has cancer. The emphasis is on the patient's perspective. Chapter 2 presents the perspectives of the doctors and nurses.

Part II covers the phase in which the patient receives first-line chemotherapy. Chapter 3 describes how patients gradually calm down and become optimistic after the existential crisis caused by the 'bad news'. Chapter 4 is about the very sick patient who doctors decide to continue treating, and the discussions that this generates among the nurses. Chapter 5 tries to find an explanation for the patient's optimism about recovery. Chapter 6 shows that in addition to optimism, patients also experience uncertainty and anxiety, and reflect on their lives.

Part III covers the recurrence of the tumour and second-line chemotherapy. Chapter 7 describes how patients realize that the cancer has metastasized, how the decision to agree to more chemotherapy develops and the feelings that this generates in the patient, his relatives and fellow patients. Chapter 8 describes how the patient's optimism gradually resides in this phase of the illness. Chapter 9 is about the patient who decides to stop treatment during third-line chemotherapy.

Part IV describes the final phase of the illness and the different ways in which patients take leave. Chapter 10 discusses the dilemmas related to the patient's optimism and their ambivalence regarding the outcome of their illness. Chapter 11 is about the patient for whom nothing more can be done, and who is sent back to his GP to die, and about the problems that this causes. This chapter also introduces the GP's perspective. Chapter 12 describes the different ways in which patients take leave and their realization of approaching death.

Part V contains the conclusions of the study. It returns to the theme of the patient's unjustified optimism. I summarize and comment on forms of communication, the ambiguous context in which treatment occurs, social influences, the slumbering realization of approaching death, the ambivalence regarding the outcome of the illness and the choice of therapy. I then compare these results with the assumptions of informed consent. Finally, in a section entitled 'The collusion' I look to the future and make some recommendations for further study.

The book concludes with an epilogue, in which relatives look back over the illness trajectory of the deceased. I then describe how I, as researcher, look back over the study. I reflect on the role, the influence and the dilemmas of the ethnographer and I describe the learning process that I experienced in my attempt to strike a balance between involvement and detachment.

PART I

Bad news and choosing therapy

1 Patients

Mr Wiersema

[10 March] 'I put the windows in this hospital,' the man in the striped pyjamas says proudly. His hand, covered in plasters, holds the stem of the wheeled trolley holding his intravenous drip. We are sitting on one of the imitation-leather sofas, separated by large indoor plants, in the hall at the front of the ward. He is in hospital because he is due to start his second course of chemotherapy.

'I've been putting windows in since I was 17,' he continues. 'Now I'm in charge. Every year I train a new group of lads. They say I can put in windows faster than anyone else in the firm. And you know what my secret is? Every morning at half past six I roll a big supply of cigarettes. Saves time later. And the wife prepares a pile of sandwiches and a flask of coffee, black coffee. When the lads and I reach the site we light a cigarette, drink a cup of coffee, eat a sandwich and draw up our plan for the day. We size things up and then get down to work. No messing around. By the end of the day the cigarettes are all finished and I go back home to the wife.

'When I've finished the chemo,' he continues as he pushes the trolley back and forth, 'I'll get back to work. You bet.' He clears his throat and says, more forcefully, 'The firm needs me. Next year I'll be back at work.'

'How did it all start?' I ask after a silence. 'How did you first notice that you were ill?'

'You need to know for your book? Well I'll tell you. One day I had a bad cold and didn't go to work. I'm hardly ever sick, you know. Then, when I went back to work a couple of weeks later, I suddenly had this pain in my chest. And I was sweating, really sweating.' He shook his head at the thought. 'That afternoon I was back at home, sick again. The wife was worried. You've met her, haven't you? She insisted that I see the doctor, and, well, she's the boss.' He winks at me conspiratorially. 'The doctor listened to my lungs and said I had bronchitis. Gave me antibiotics. When I'd finished them I still wasn't better so I went back for more. This time he also gave me prednisone. But nothing seemed to help, so he sent me to the hospital for further tests.

'Here they really gave me a thorough going over. They made X-rays of my lungs, and the doctor said he could see a *mass*, a mass that didn't belong there. Doesn't sound too good, I said. So they had a look inside through a tube. Horrible, I could hardly breathe. They told us to come for the results a couple of days later and, well, you were there so you know the rest.'

Bad news and the choice of treatment

[8 February, 9:30 am] The lung specialists Guido Liem, Ronald Veerman and Marcel Heller and the research fellow Dorien Meulman have been discussing the patients who were expected at the outpatient clinic this morning. When they have left Dr Liem's office he buttons up his white coat and takes a file from the pile on his desk. 'Our first patient this morning is Mr Wiersema,' he tells me. 'Last week we did some tests and it appears he had a small-cell lung carcinoma with metastases in the liver. I have to break the news to him, and that is always difficult.' He gets up and goes to call Mr Wiersema from the waiting room.

'Please sit down,' Dr Liem tells Mr and Mrs Wiersema when they enter the office. 'You've already met Mrs The, haven't you? She'll be joining us again today, if you don't mind.' He sits down at his desk, Mr Wiersema's open file in front of him. Mr Wiersema is clearly uncomfortable, Mrs Wiersema looks worried. She does not participate in the discussion. Mr Wiersema discusses with the doctor, alternating between anxiously avoiding Dr Liem's gaze, cracking jokes and speculating about the future. I will always remember him like that.

'We discussed the various issues last time,' Dr Liem says. 'I'll show you on the X-rays what it is we're worried about.' He walks around the desk and stands next to the light box. 'You see that white patch there?' He points to the X-ray. 'It shouldn't be there. The question now is, what is it? I told you last time that we were worried it might be malignant, but I didn't want to be premature. We did the bronchoscopy and the CT scan and now I have the results.' Dr Liem returns to his chair. 'I'm, afraid,' he continues, 'that I've got bad news for you.' Mrs Wiersema closes her eyes. Mr Wiersema leans his elbow on the edge of the desk, covers his eyes with his hand takes a deep breath. 'You have a small-cell lung carcinoma,' Dr Liem continues. 'Or, in other words, lung cancer.' There is silence. Mrs Wiersema looks at her husband.

'You're probably wondering if anything can be done,' Dr Liem resumes, trying to fill the silence. Mr Wiersema watches the doctor, following his every gesture. 'Well something can be done. I'll explain. I would prefer to recommend you for an operation, in which case we would just remove the tumour and that would be the end of that. But unfortunately we can't operate in your case because the tumour is right next to the jugular vein. The second option is to do nothing and see what happens.'

'But then the tumour will continue to grow,' says Mr Wiersema, his gaze focused on the doctor.

'Yes, then the tumour would continue to grow,' Dr Liem nods. The third option is chemotherapy, and that's what I want to discuss with you. But let me start by saying that I don't think that I can make you better. The type of tumour you have is very aggressive. It grows rapidly and spreads easily. The chance of cure is very small, about 7 per cent. But, if you want us to, we can do something for you. We can give you chemotherapy. This type of tumour is generally responsive to chemotherapy.'

Mr Wiersema draws a deep breath.

'If you agree you would be admitted to the ward for five days every three weeks to receive the treatment. In the intervening period you would come to the outpatient clinic once a week for check-ups, blood tests and X-rays.'

'What can we expect from the treatment, doctor?' asks Mrs Wiersema.

'You have to look at it like this,' Dr Liem answers. 'If we don't do anything then the end could come very soon. Your husband would no longer be with us in two or three months. With chemotherapy his chances are much better. The advantage of chemotherapy, if I may put it that way, is that it spreads throughout the body. So if the tumour has already spread and there are other small tumours that we can't see yet, then the chemotherapy will eradicate them.' The couple nod.

'The unpleasant thing about this tumour is that it is very persistent and it tends to come back after treatment. If the therapy does not seem to have any effect then we will stop immediately, because that won't benefit you at all. In that case we would have to evaluate the situation again. You have to prepare yourself for both good and bad news in the weeks to come.

'It's unbelievable, Mr Wiersema says. 'I don't feel sick at all. Next year I'll be 50, and I'm never sick. I'm tired and I cough a bit, that's all. It's unbelievable.'

'He has a bit of flu,' Mrs Wiersema chips in.

'Really,' says Dr Liem. 'Chemotherapy has disadvantages that you should know about,' he continues. 'It can make you nauseous, but we can give you something for that. You will lose your hair. You'll have to come to the hospital regularly for treatment and check-ups. You have to realize that it is something you will have to persevere with.'

'We've achieved good results with the kind of therapy I'm offering you, and we're planning to make more use of it in the future. But before we can do that we need to prove scientifically that it really works. That sounds complicated, but what it means is that we give that treatment to a group of patients and closely monitor what the effect is by doing various tests. I'm sure you'd want to know exactly how the treatment was working. What do you think? Do you want some time to think it over? Are there any questions?'

'Doctor, we'll take whatever we are offered,' Mr Wiersema answers resolutely. 'If we don't, we'll only regret it later. We don't need to think about anything, we'll do it.'

'Good,' the doctor nods. 'I've got a form here with everything that I've just told you. You can take it home to read. If you are going to participate then we'll need a signature.' Dr Liem points to the dotted line on the bottom of the form. 'You can bring it along next time. The important point is that everything has been explained to you properly.'

'Would you do it if it were you, doctor?' Mr Wiersema asks as he signs the form.

'Yes,' Dr Liem answers seriously. 'I'd try it. And I think we should get started as soon as possible.'

'Do you think I have a chance?' asks Mr Wiersema.

'Of course, otherwise I wouldn't suggest therapy.'

Not feeling sick

I started with Mr Wiersema's bad news interview because it was characteristic of most such interviews. It is a blueprint for the bad news interview that I became familiar with during my years in the Ruysdael Clinic. Only the odd junior doctor deviated from this pattern. Differences between the interviews were caused primarily by the patients and depended on factors such as the physical condition of the patient and whether or not he questioned the doctor. In this chapter I describe variations on the bad news interview. Most patients with a small-cell lung carcinoma – like Mr Wiersema – do not feel seriously ill, and certainly not *fatally* ill, at the time of diagnosis. Symptoms are generally described as a persistent flu. Patients generally take into account the possibility that something more is wrong than simply flu, but they are certainly not expecting a death sentence. This takes most patients completely by surprise. Medical technology is far ahead of the patient's own body in making the diagnosis (Kellehear 1992: 83). For patients who still feel relatively healthy, the news that they could be dead in two or three months is totally incomprehensible. Being unable to trust their own senses makes patients uncertain and gives them the feeling of being alienated from their bodies. The measure of 'how well they are' is, from this point on, no longer how they feel but the results of laboratory tests and X-rays, and the interpretations that the doctors attach to these. As one patient put it during a bad news interview, 'It's the X-rays that tell me that I'm sick, not my body.'

Truth and patterns of disclosure

Unlike in the recent past, doctors nowadays inform patients that they are terminally ill. Studies from the 1960s have shown that doctors withheld the prognosis because they thought that patients would not be able to cope with the knowledge.[1] And there are some poignant examples from literature as well (Solzehnitsyn 1968). In the 1970s there was a change and research from 1979 shows that, by then, 90 per cent of doctors reported telling patients the truth (Novack et al. 1979). A more recent study has shown that currently the vast majority of cancer patients want to be informed about diagnosis and treatment (Richards et al. 1995: 113). Patients consider that they have a right to know.[2] Here I would like to note that there can be a discrepancy between, on the one hand, how doctors *say* they act (and indeed think they act) and what they actually do (see McIntosh 1974; van Busschbach 1986; Verhaak et al. 1986), and on the other hand how patients interpret their actions. This discrepancy will be described in detail and analysed in Part II.

What is the pattern of disclosure in the bad news interview? Generally speaking the interview consists of two parts: first the doctor tells the patient the bad news, and second he discusses the various treatment options with the patient. The patient has generally already been prepared for the bad news in earlier discussions. For example, Mr Wiersema came to the lung specialist with complaints. During the first consultation an illness history was taken, tests were carried out and X-rays were made. The X-rays revealed lesions, which in turn made further tests necessary. At this point the doctor already suspected cancer and told Mr Wiersema as much. 'What could the patch on the X-ray mean? It could be an infection, but then you should have responded to the antibiotics. It could also be – and now I'm considering the worst scenario – cancer. But we'll need to do more tests to find out what it really is.' In this way the bad news is presented to the patient in phases. When the final test results have been received, the patient is informed of the definitive diagnosis. What this usually means is that the doctor's initial suspicions are confirmed. I refer to the formal discussion in which the doctor presents the definitive diagnosis to the patient as the bad news interview.

In the bad news interview, in addition to informing the patient that he has lung cancer, the doctor also informs him what kind of tumour it is and that he is incurably ill. This hard reality is presented as softly as possible. I never heard a doctor say 'you are going to die soon,' or 'this is the end of the road'. They said things like, 'I don't think I'm going to be able to cure you', or, 'the chance of a cure is very slim, only 7 per cent'. This is followed almost immediately by the doctor asking, rhetorically, what can be done. With this question the first part of the interview, in which the bad news

---

1 Research by Oken (1961) shows that 95 per cent of specialists did not inform their patients of the diagnosis. Glaser and Strauss (1965) report a similar situation.
2 Rampen and van Dam (1987: 508) report that patients think they have a right to be told the diagnosis.

is revealed passes over smoothly into the second part that is all about treatment.

Usually the doctor begins by describing three treatment options. First, surgery, although this is usually not an option as the tumour has often spread or is situated in an area that makes surgery impossible. In fact, as Dr Liem explains in the next chapter, surgery is almost never a real option in the case of small-cell lung carcinoma. It is mentioned more in the way of explaining why it is not an option. The second option is 'do nothing and see what happens,' which in practice means letting the tumour develop further with the patient usually dying within three months. Hardly any patients seriously consider this option. During almost five years in the Ruysdael Clinic I only met three patients who deliberately refused treatment.[3] I discuss these in the next chapter. Chemotherapy then remains as the third and obvious option. The standard therapy for non-small-cell lung carcinoma, radiation therapy, is not mentioned. In describing the advantage of chemotherapy ('it gets to *every corner* of the body, so *just in case* there is a metastasis hiding somewhere, the chemo will get it') the doctor gives the reason for this: radiation therapy is local whereas small-cell lung carcinomas have often metastasized.

A number of important issues are concentrated in the brief space of the bad news interview: the bad news is passed on, treatment options are discussed and a choice of therapy is made. Quite often the patient commences treatment on the very same day. For this reason, the bad news interview has been referred to as a 'marathon session'.[4] As a result of this marathon character, the patient hardly has time to digest the bad news and consider the options properly.[5] As a result, we may wonder to what extent the patient's decisions about treatment are really 'well-considered'.

It is not only the concentration of emotionally charged information in such a short time span that makes it difficult for patients to fully understand what is happening. The content of that information is also equivocal. First, the doctor shocks the patient by telling him that there is a very serious problem. He then mitigates this by saying that 'something can be done'. In the dual grip of fear and hope, the patient commences chemotherapy.[6]

---

3 In the Ruysdael Clinic there are 200 new cases of lung cancer annually, a quarter of whom have small-cell lung carcinoma.

4 The term is taken from Siminoff et al. (1989). The consultations described by Siminoff et al. were more extensive than the ones I observed, and included physical examinations and anamnesis which, in the case of this study, had taken place earlier. However, because so many important issues were discussed and important decisions made in the bad news interviews described here, I think the term is appropriate here as well.

5 Fallowfield et al. (1986) refer to this as 'picking up the pieces'.

6 This section is based on de Swaan 1985: 18–19.

Meeting Mr Dekker

[7 February, 9:15 am] I hurry down the corridor carrying a pile of clean sheets and pillowcases, on my way to make the beds on the ward. As I pass the single rooms I catch a glimpse of a large, heavily built man of about 50, leaning over a table and examining something through a magnifying glass. I stop and see that he is painting a small tin soldier.

When I pass the room again in the afternoon and glance in, he just happens to look up from his painting. He gives me a friendly nod. I stop in the doorway. 'I wondered what you were doing,' I say. He turns the soldier toward me and then points to the window sill, on which a whole army is lined up.

'Very nice,' I say, walking over to the window sill to examine them. 'You're skilled with a fine brush.'

'It takes concentration, and that keeps me calm,' he explains. 'That's why I started. Three years ago I had a stomach ulcer and I had to take things easy. "Relax," the doctor said. But that wasn't easy for me. I can't just sit still, I need to be active. So one day my wife said, "why don't you have a hobby? Then you won't have time to worry about other things." At first I didn't think it was such a good idea. But later I thought, "Why not try it?" I used to have a few soldiers, and I thought they were wonderful, but I didn't have the money for a whole army. Just look at me, I've become a boy again.' He taps his brush on the saucer on which he has been mixing paint. 'The days here in the hospital are long,' he continues. 'The *waiting* is long,' he adds. 'They think I've got cancer. That doctor, Dr Kooiman, the one who did the test.' He points to his nose and then lets his finger slide down along his windpipe to his lungs. 'The test with the pipe through my nose, the bigro . . . er, the bigroscopy . . .'

'Bronchoscopy?'

'Exactly. That doctor said that he had to wait for the results from the lab, but that he was almost certain that it was cancer that he had seen in my lungs. Tomorrow or the day after they should know for certain exactly what it is. I already knew that something was wrong. I suspected something, but there was the uncertainty of not knowing for sure.'

'Let me introduce myself,' I say. 'I haven't done that yet. I'm Anne-Mei The.' I hold out my hand.

'And I'm Klaas Dekker.' A firm handshake.

'I look like a nurse, but actually I'm not,' I explain. 'I work for the university and I'm doing a study of how doctors, nurses and patients talk to each other in the hospital. I'm interested in how information is provided, how things are discussed, how decisions are made and what the various parties think about this. I'm wearing these,' I point to my white trousers, blue and white striped T-shirt and plimsolls, 'to be as inconspicuous as possible. I want the things I see to be as normal as possible, as though I wasn't here.'

'But you *are* here,' Mr Dekker says, his eyes laughing.

'Yes, I am,' I admit.

'So you talk to everyone?' he asks, looking at me questioningly.

'Yes,' I nod. 'At least, if they agree. I talk to people and I observe what they are doing. And I'm going to write a book about it.'

I am interrupted by voices outside the room. A young woman enters with a little girl of about ten.

'My nieces, Vera and Roosje.' Mr Dekker introduces me and we shake hands.

'If that's okay with you, I'd like to come back later,' I say.

'That's fine,' he answers and waves his hand. 'Any time.'

The little girl climbs onto his lap.

[9 February, morning] Mr Dekker moves to a bigger room with five other patients. One of my jobs is to help the nurse responsible for this room to wash patients and make beds. I also accompany the doctor on his rounds. Whenever I pass, Mr Dekker gives me a friendly nod. At the end of the day I see him in the common room reading the newspaper. When I enter he raises his hand in greeting.

'Have a few minutes off?' he asks, initiating conversation.

'Well, in fact, I came to ask how you were doing,' I explain.

'Okay, I'm okay. As you heard this morning during rounds, Dr Kooiman is going to talk to us this afternoon. My wife and Johan, our stepson, are coming, and then we're going to talk. And I have to admit that I'm looking forward to it.'

I sit down next to him.

'The waiting is terrible,' he says.

'I can imagine,' I say. There is a long silence. 'Mr Dekker,' I resume, 'I would like to talk to you about your experiences here in the hospital and at home. I am interested personally, but also for my work.'

'For your book?' he asks.

'Yes, for my book. But also for the people who will read it. It might be useful for other patients who are in the same situation as yourself. I think it would also be useful for doctors and nurses to understand what you are experiencing. But you needn't feel obliged. You should only agree if you want to.'

There is a twinkle in his eye. 'Don't worry,' he says, 'it's okay.'

Mr Dekker kept his problem hidden from his wife

'It's a long story,' Mr Dekker clears his throat. 'In fact it's my wife's fault that I waited so long. She had a bad car accident eight years ago. It affected her eyesight and she's had bad backache ever since. Her younger sister was with her in the car and she . . . she was killed instantly. My brother-in-law had gone off to Germany suddenly a year before. Wanted to make a new start. My sister-in-law didn't want anything more to do with him. She managed to get an injunction preventing him from seeing the children. So after the accident the children had nobody. We adopted the three youngest ones. You saw the girls here the other day. The boy, Johan, is coming this afternoon. We don't have any children of our own. We wanted children but we couldn't have any. Now we have three. We're very fond of them, and they of us. But that accident is a source of great sadness.

'Rietje, my wife, can't do all the things she used to. Domestic chores are too much. In fact, everything is too much. She has terrible nightmares. She has flashbacks of the accident. But the worst thing is that she has changed. She used to be merry and enjoy life. Now everything is too much effort.

'And you know, I feel guilty,' he says, and falls silent. 'I was supposed to accompany them that evening.' He stares at the wall. They were going to visit their other sister, but I don't get on with her. I wasn't in the mood for a whole evening with her, so I said "Why don't you go alone?" If I'd have gone with them it might not have happened. At the time Rietje hadn't had her driving licence that long and hadn't much driving experience.' He falls silent and clenches his fists. 'Rietje says it's not my fault, but I still feel guilty. I could have gone with her but I didn't feel like it.' The newspaper on his lap falls to the floor.

'Since that accident I've tried to cushion her against unpleasant things, tried to make her more merry. I don't want her to worry about me. That's why I didn't tell her about my problem. At first I thought I just had a persistent cold. I was always tired and had a bad cough. I had difficulty breathing and had a heavy feeling in my chest. That's when I stopped smoking. That reduced the coughing, but the heavy feeling in the chest and the fatigue remained.

'I didn't tell my wife anything. I didn't want to burden her, I didn't want her to worry. During the day, when I was at work, I could keep it hidden. But in the evening, at home, it was more difficult. So straight after dinner I used to go up to the loft, where I have old televisions and stereos that I repair. 'I'm going up to my repairs,' I used to say.

'But all I did was sit behind the workbench worrying. Something was wrong; I was sure of that. But how wrong? I kept thinking: If things are really going wrong, what will happen to her and the kids? Then the moment came that I couldn't avoid it any longer. I'm a chimney sweep and one day, when I came down from the roof and needed a quarter of an hour to get my breath before I could talk to the customer, I realized that I had to stop denying. I went to the doctor and asked him to refer me to the hospital. I'd been to see him a couple of weeks before, but he said that there was nothing seriously wrong. So I went to the hospital. That was last week. They made X-rays of my lungs and I was admitted while they did other tests.'

Bad news and the choice for treatment

[9 February, pm]. At three o'clock sharp Mr Dekker and his wife are seated next to each other in the coffee lounge. Next to them is their stepson, Johan, a young man in his early 20s. Opposite are Karin de Boer, a nurse, and me. I had Mr and Mrs Dekker's permission to attend. Karin has just put a tray of coffee on the low table between us. There is a clinking of spoons on cups, but otherwise there is silence, a heavy silence. The atmosphere is tense. Dr Kooiman arrives and shakes hands with Mr and Mrs Dekker.

'We've already discussed some of the issues,' Dr Kooiman says, nodding in the direction of Mr Dekker. 'After the bronchoscopy.'

Mr Dekker nods affirmatively, his gaze focused on the doctor.

'I said at the time that I was reasonably sure that there was a tumour in your lung. I'm afraid that the laboratory tests have confirmed that you have cancer.' Dr Kooiman is silent for a few moments, his face serious, Mr Dekker closes his eyes.

'How long have I got, doctor?' he asks in a subdued voice, his eyes still closed.

'That's difficult to say at this point,' Dr Kooiman answers. 'It depends on so many things, such as how you respond to treatment. We'll have to wait and see how things develop before I can say anything meaningful about that.'

'But you can give me *some* idea, can't you?'

'That would be very general, though, and I don't want you focusing too much on a date like that. It would be like having to pass a death sentence; like saying: you are going to die on such-and-such a date.'

'But is it a question of weeks, months?'

'No, that's not the way to look at it,' Dr Kooiman responds resolutely. If we give you chemotherapy you should think in terms of *years*.'

Mr Dekker hits his right fist into his left palm. 'Damn it!' He leans forward, elbows on the table, head in his hands. Tears spring into Mrs Dekker's eyes. She puts her hand on his arm. 'Let yourself go, Klaas, it's okay to cry sometimes,' she says.

'Just leave me alone for a minute,' he answers. Then he looks up at the doctor. 'So I'm not going to die straight away?' he asks, his tone pleading.

'No.' Dr Kooiman shakes his head. 'There's no reason at all to think like that now.' He sounds reassuring.

'I was so worried, doctor,' Mr Dekker admits. 'I was just *so* worried that this was the end; that I wouldn't be here in a few weeks, months.' He breathes in deeply.

'The kind of lung cancer that you have is very aggressive,' Dr Kooiman explains. 'It grows very rapidly. On the other hand – and that is an advantage, if I might say so – this form of cancer is also very sensitive to chemotherapy; it can be treated. We can offer you a course of chemotherapy, and I would strongly advise you to accept, because if we do nothing then the end will come very quickly. In two, three months that could be it.' Dr Kooiman pauses for a while. 'At the moment we don't know whether the tumour has spread to other parts of the body. We need to investigate that further. I can tell you that we have found malignant cells in the lymph nodes. But that doesn't make any difference for chemotherapy; the treatment remains the same. The advantage of chemotherapy is that it gets into every corner of the body. It not only gets to the tumour in the lungs, but it also gets to metastases if there are any in other parts of the body.'

'I'll try anything,' Mr Dekker interrupts. '*Anything*. I can't leave her behind.' It is a cry of despair. Mrs Dekker bites her bottom lip. Johan stares out of the window, chewing obstinately on his chewing gum.

'We're going to tackle this together,' Dr Kooiman says encouragingly. 'You have to have courage.' Mr Dekker nods.

'Now I must tell you a few things about the treatment,' Dr Kooiman continues. 'Chemotherapy has a number of side effects. Your hair will drop out . . .'

'I don't care about that,' Mr Dekker interrupts.

'But it will grow again afterwards. And you might be nauseous, but we can give you medication for that. Chemotherapy has an effect on your blood, and before we start with the next course of therapy we must make sure that your blood has recovered fully from the previous course. We check your blood regularly.'

'Doctor, will I lose weight and become so thin? Mrs Westra in the next bed also has lung cancer, and she's really emaciated.'

'Not necessarily,' says Dr Kooiman. 'It depends. You need to make sure that you eat well during the treatment. The treatment consists of five courses and each course consists of three infusions of chemotherapy. During the first course you will get infusions on three consecutive days. Then you have a three-week break and then another three days of chemotherapy. You'll need to be admitted to the hospital for this. We've had good results with this therapy. They've done a lot of research, especially in America. So we know that it works, but we need to prove it. That means that we have to give the treatment to a group of patients and then see how it works. We do that by testing the blood, making X-rays and doing various other tests. So the treatment is part of a research project. It's all described here in this information leaflet. You can take it home and read it at your leisure.'

Mr Dekker nods.

'If you are interested in participating then we would like you to put your signature at the bottom of this form. You can take the form with you and bring it back next time.'

Mr Dekker asks his wife for a pen and signs the form. 'I don't need to think about that,' he says, and hands the form back to the doctor.

'When can I start?' he asks. 'Today?'

'So you want the therapy?' Dr Kooiman asks.

'Do I have any choice, doctor?' Mr Dekker asks. 'No I don't, do I?'

Dr Kooiman shakes his head slowly.

'I'm standing with my back to the wall, and I don't want to waste any time.'

'I'll try and arrange for you to start the first course tomorrow. With this type of tumour it's important to lose as little time as possible. Do you have any questions?' Dr Kooiman looks round the table at the other participants.

'We have a problem with the GP,' Mrs Dekker says. 'He waited too long before referring my husband to the hospital, Klaas ended up asking to be referred himself. And now . . .' Her voice breaks. 'Now that things have turned out badly he's nowhere to be seen. I think that's terrible.'

Dr Kooiman nods understandingly. 'Unpleasant,' he says. 'But there's not much I can do about that now. I think it would be good to go and discuss it with him.' He stands up, signalling the end of the meeting.

'And you can always come to us if you have questions,' he adds. We have an outpatient clinic three times a week. You won't be seeing me there though, you'll see Dr Heller, Dr Liem and Dr Veerman. They have specialized in lung cancer.' He shakes hands round the table and leaves the room.

Later Karin de Boer says to me, 'I like Menno Kooiman's way of dealing with patients. He tackles the issue head-on, and that helps the patient. It's no use simply being negative about it. Menno's always very involved with the patient. He's one of the few doctors who takes time during rounds to sit down next to the bed so that he can talk to the patient on the same level. I've seen him reading his paper in the room of a patient who didn't like to be alone.

'Mr Dekker was almost begging for therapy,' she continues. And what could be nicer than granting him his wish?'

Prognosis

There are a number of differences between the bad news interviews of Mr Wiersema and Mr Dekker. Mr Dekker's interview took place on the ward rather than in the outpatient department. A small proportion of patients receives the diagnosis while they are in hospital undergoing tests. Both patients had been prepared for the bad news beforehand by the doctor and both were given the information in stages. The most obvious difference between the two settings is the presence of a nurse during interviews on the ward. When nurses are present it is mainly in order to keep the nursing staff informed of decisions; it is exclusively the doctors who provide the information.[7] When nurses have *participated* in the interview it makes it much easier for them to clarify various issues for the patient later. The presence of a nurse also usually provides extra emotional support for the patient and his relatives. After Dr Kooiman had left, Karin de Boer remained behind to talk to the Dekkers. Her role was not informative; it gave them the opportunity to let off steam and express what was really troubling them. All those involved in this study admitted the importance of having nurses involved in bad news interviews, but in practice there were various reasons why nurses were often not present. For example, doctors may forget to invite them, or they may be too busy to attend.

Mr Dekker was one of the few patients in this study who realized that they had a fatal illness. This is partly because he felt sick, much sicker than

---

7 In a year-long study in the intensive care department of a different hospital, I noticed that there the nurses did participate in the bad news interviews. The doctor would initiate the discussion but the nurses would chip in as and when they thought this was necessary.

Mr Wiersema, for example. His symptoms – a grossly swollen lymph node in the neck and shortness of breath – worried him because he associated them with cancer (Kellehear 1992: 83–4). Apparently patients who have symptoms of this illness are seldom surprised when they hear that they have cancer and are going to die (Wagener 1987: 1106). Mr Dekker's anticipation may also have derived from something I have already mentioned relating to his biography: the realization that life was finite.

Mr Dekker anticipated the truth, and when he finally decided to go for tests he wanted to know what his prospects were. To a certain extent he was happy that the bad news interview brought the uncertainty to an end. Patients claim that this first phase, when they are waiting for the diagnosis, is the most stressful of all. Not knowing gives rise to fear and anxiety, and many patients feel an acute need for more information. Once the diagnosis has been revealed, they can try to establish a new equilibrium and gain control over their illness (Regt et al. 1998: 10).

In Mr Wiersema's bad news interview, Dr Liem said that without treatment he had about two to three months to live. The doctor provided this information *actively*, by which I mean he *volunteered* information about the patient's prognosis without treatment. He was, however, vague about the prognosis with treatment. He said, 'It would improve your chances significantly,' without explaining what a 'significant improvement' meant. In most of the bad news interviews I observed doctors did not actively inform patients how much time they had left. That doctors avoid discussing prognosis, or neutralize it, is well known (Costain Schou 1993: 239). It is also known that they tend to shift attention to treatment. Mr Wiersema was, like most patients, satisfied with the information provided and did not ask any further questions. Mr Dekker was not. He repeatedly asked Dr Kooiman about his prognosis. Dr Kooiman simply answered that he would be able to say more later on. He placed Mr Dekker's future in the context of the treatment: further prognosis is only possible after the results of further tests have been received (de Swaan 1985). When Mr Dekker insisted, Dr Kooiman gave a careful but optimistic indication: 'You should think in terms of *years*' (de Swaan 1985).

To some extent, doctors adjust what they say to what the patients ask them, for example in giving the prognosis. The rule is that patients have to ask for information. When they do not, this is interpreted as not wanting to know. To a certain extent, this is a correct interpretation. Early in the study I was surprised by patients' passive attitude to their prognosis. The social distance between doctor and patient is often large. Doctors have degrees and often represent a world that patients look up to. This may make it difficult for patients to demand information on what is important for them (The 1997a, 1998). Another explanation is that patients do not want to be difficult and waste the doctor's time (Regt et al. 1998: 24). During the course of the study I noticed that it was not just a question of having courage to ask that made patients passive, but also fear of what the answer might be (de Swaan 1985: 36).

Patients' narratives

I have described the first interview with Mr Dekker in some detail because it gives some idea of his life before the illness. It also illustrates how his life and the lives of his family are interwoven. Mr Dekker talks emotionally about how his illness affects his life and the lives of his closest family (Gelauff and Manschot 1997: 195). A serious illness with a disastrous outcome affects not only the patient – who has to achieve closure – but also propels his family into a period of transition – they will have to find a new equilibrium without a husband and stepfather (Finch and Wallis 1993: 53–6).

The classic sociological studies of death focus on dying and its rituals, symbols and psychological phases (Glaser and Strauss 1965; Sudnow 1967; Kübler-Ross 1969). This is important, but not the whole story. Individuals who are confronted with death are influenced by their life histories and their relationships with others (Finch and Wallis 1993). In the literature on the life cycle, it is surprising how little attention is given to dying. The central significance of dying as a phase in the life cycle is that people can anticipate it. In fact, it is the only phase that can be anticipated with certainty. Although everyone knows they are going to die, they only start thinking about it seriously when the time comes. Growing old, the loss of loved ones and illness serve to bring the realization of mortality closer. The 'advantage', if I may use the term, of illnesses like small-cell lung carcinoma compared with acutely fatal diseases like heart attacks, is that patients have the chance to reflect on the consequences of their death for those around them and have the chance to prepare and say goodbye to loved ones. They are, in other words, able to achieve satisfactory closure. Ideally, medical treatment could be tailored individually to each patient. Those who need time to complete unfinished business could choose life-extending treatment, whereas those who do not think that the side effects of treatment are worth the extra few months of life, or who cannot cope with the numbing wait for death, could choose not to extend the final phase. In an era in which individual autonomy dominates and patients' right of self-determination is anchored in law, the patients in this study are able to shape their own final phase of life.

How patients cope depends on the individual involved. Mr Dekker is different to Mr Wiersema, and in this book it will become clear how they each give form to the final phase. This depends on personality, attitude to life and biography. Mr Dekker's life story is not simply meant to add descriptive colour; it is important because the final phase of that story is played out in the hospital. His experiences throughout his life play a role in determining how he copes with his illness, how he interacts with doctors, and how he decides about treatment options.

Mr Dekker's particular family situation influences the way he responds to his illness. He tries to protect his wife by hiding his symptoms from her. He believes that a man is responsible for his family, and this is reinforced after his wife's accident. This is partly because he has to do more (his wife cannot do as much as before and there are three children to take care of) and partly because he feels guilty about her accident. The fact that he interpreted his symptoms as a sign of something incurable even before he had consulted a doctor (he wept and told his wife this would be their last Christmas together) is undoubtedly also related to guilt about the accident. In a later stage of his illness he remarked that the accident had taken away completely the assumption of invulnerability, the idea that it was only others who were touched by fate.

So I do not present Mr Dekker's life story as *couleur locale*, but because it is a good example of the changes that can occur in a patient's life and the way in which they bear on his illness. It illustrates what is important in Mr Dekker's life, and in particular what is important for him in the final phase of life. It is these (non-medical) factors that play an important role in whether or not patients decide to accept life-extending therapy. Mr Dekker was worried about his wife and stepchildren. He needed more time to help them plan their future. This would enable him to make the necessary financial arrangements. More time would also have given his wife and stepchildren the opportunity to talk about and prepare for his death. Personal factors like these can be very important for patients, and they should have a place in the discussions about therapy.

Intermezzo: meeting

Although I describe the methodological aspects of this study in detail, I want to say something here about the way in which I present my material, how I was introduced to patients and the informed consent procedure. By presenting my data in the form of narrative and dialogue, in which the researcher is also present, I hope to achieve a degree of transparency; to show the reader how I participated in hospital life, how I collected data and how I interpreted it. The description of my meeting with Mr Dekker is intended to illustrate how I came into contact with patients, explained what I was doing and asked them to participate in the study.

On the ward I automatically came into contact with patients because I was working with the nurses. Sometimes the doctors and nurses 'tipped me off' that a patient who might be interesting for my study was about to be admitted. In most cases, as with Mr Dekker, I first approached them for an informal conversation. Sometimes nurses introduced me. In the outpatient department I was introduced by the doctor and followed that up later with a meeting in which I explained to the patient in more detail what I wanted to do.

In all cases my introduction to the patients was in phases; at each meeting I told them more about the study. It was a question of adequately judging the situation and interpreting the response. If patients appeared to be uninterested or if it was difficult to establish rapport, then I did not pursue the matter; if we got on well and they took the initiative to come and chat with me, then I kept visiting them. In this way my contact with the participants in this study developed 'naturally' and in the course of time I had built up a group of 30 patients.

Mr Heuvel's bad news interview

[1 April] 'Mr Heuvel, born in 1927, referred from Internal Medicine,' Dr Liem reads from the file. 'Dr Jaspers writes that the patient consulted his GP three weeks ago because he was nauseous. He was then admitted.' The doctor's voice drones on, as he follows the text with his finger, 'a malignant process originating in the lungs, possibly a small-cell lung carcinoma with a massive metastasis in the liver, which is the cause of the current complaint.' He looks up from the file. 'We'll have to do some additional tests to be sure of the diagnosis. And a bronchoscopy, preferably today, so we can start chemotherapy on Monday. He might be suitable for the trial. We'll have to discuss with him and see if he agrees.'

Dr Liem gets up and goes out into the waiting room. A few minutes later he comes back, pushing a man in a wheelchair. The man is so ill that he slouches in the chair. Dr Liem's expression is serious. When I catch his eye he shakes his head. Following them is a woman, with a large handbag in one hand and a wrinkled-up handkerchief in the other. Her eyes are red and she looks around the room anxiously. The doctor parks the wheelchair in front of his desk and puts on the brake. He drags over a chair for Mrs Heuvel. She sits down, her large handbag on her lap. Dr Liem takes his place behind the desk. I sit next to him on a stool. He leans forward toward the patient.

'Mr Heuvel,' he says, in a calm voice, 'can you tell me what is wrong?'

'I've got . . .' Mr Heuvel's voice breaks and he sags further in his wheelchair. There is sweat on his forehead and his skin is yellow.

'He's got terrible stomach ache,' Mrs Heuvel says, as she fiddles with her handbag. Mr Heuvel's stomach is swollen; it strains against the buttons of his shirt. 'He was a bit nauseous,' Mrs Heuvel continues, 'but it's become much worse. He doesn't enjoy his food any more. I've tried everything, minced meat, salads.' She is talking faster now. 'I cycled to town every day for those salads. I thought that would be the right thing for him to eat when he wasn't feeling well. He'd start off okay, but after one spoonful he'd had enough. Then my daughter said that what he needed was dairy products. So then I gave him yoghurt, curds, muesli . . .'

'Lack of appetite,' Dr Liem summarizes on the form in front of him.

'He can't keep anything in. He's hardly eaten a thing in the last four weeks.'

'Nauseous,' I read on Dr Liem's form.

'I've tried everything. I've minced his food,' the stream of words continues. 'But you don't want to go straight to the doctor. That's how we were brought up, not to complain. You don't want to moan. But after a few weeks I said, "This isn't normal; you have to go to the doctor."' Mr Heuvel is sweating profusely. His eyes are closed and he is rocking gently from side to side.

'What does your husband do during the day?' Dr Liem asks.

'Nothing. I keep telling him to get out of bed. I have to call him, otherwise he would just stay there. When he comes down stairs he installs himself on the sofa and falls asleep. Then he falls to one side.' She illustrates by leaning over to the left. 'Then I wake him up and he sits straight, but after a while he falls asleep again and falls over to the other side.' She leans to the right. 'All he does is sleep.'

Dr Liem nods. 'I would like to examine you,' he says to Mr Heuvel, who straightens himself and slowly stands up. His breathing is heavy as he waddles to the examination table. Twice I think he is going to fall and jump up to assist him, but he manages to reach the table. Mrs Heuvel follows him and helps him undress. (Later Dr Liem told me that he had not assisted Mr Heuvel because he wanted to see whether he was capable of walking by himself). After the examination, Dr Liem once again examines the X-rays on the viewing box. He then replaces them with a CT scan.

'He's never been like this before,' Mrs Heuvel resumes. 'I told him he had to eat something otherwise he'd weaken, and that's not good . . .'

'There's something I must tell you,' Dr Liem interrupts her. He puts his pen down and looks at Mr Heuvel. 'You are seriously ill,' he says. 'And I want to admit you to hospital immediately.' Mr Heuvel appears not to be listening.

'I'd hoped you would,' Mrs Heuvel responds. She sounds relieved.

'Madam, your husband is very sick,' says Dr Liem.

Mrs Heuvel hides her face in her hands and a shock goes through her body.

'I'm sorry to have to tell you,' Dr Liem continues, 'but you need to know. He has a tumour in his lung and it has spread to his liver. It's the tumour in the liver that's causing his current problems. The only thing we can do for him is to try chemotherapy. That will make him feel even worse for a while. We'll have to make him sicker in order to reduce the tumour, if I may put it like that.'

Mrs Heuvel is crying. 'I knew it, I knew it,' she says. 'When we were referred to *this* outpatient clinic I knew it must be cancer.'

'What do you think, Mr Heuvel?' Dr Liem focuses on the patient again. Mr Heuvel shrugs. His eyelids droop. He seems indifferent.

'We need to start the treatment today. If we don't, then you don't have long to go. And I have to tell you honestly that I'm not sure whether the treatment will help. There's no time to lose. What do you think?' He looks at Mrs Heuvel.

She looks helplessly at Dr Liem, then at her husband, who appears oblivious to the exchange, and then back at Dr Liem.

'Shall we try it?' Dr Liem asks.

'Yes,' she answers. 'You're the doctor.' She shrugs in despair. 'If you think that's best . . .' Her voice fades. She wipes her eyes with her handkerchief.

'I'll call the ward and tell them you're on your way,' Dr Liem says, terminating the interview. As he says goodbye to Mrs Heuvel, still in tears, he puts his hand on her shoulder. 'I'll inform your GP,' he says.

When Mr and Mrs Heuvel have left Dr Liem says, 'You're probably wondering why I didn't say anything more about the trial. That's because he's too sick. He wouldn't be able to cope with all the tests. He needs immediate treatment, otherwise it will be too late.'

The reason for Mr Heuvel not being included in the trial had, in fact, not crossed my mind; I had been much too occupied with the performance I had been witnessing.

Dr Liem picks up the phone. 'Guido Liem, Ruysdael Clinic, Department of Lung Diseases,' he says. I've just had one of your patients, Mr Heuvel, in my outpatient clinic.

. . .

'Yes, it took a while for us to reach a diagnosis.'

. . .

'A small-cell lung carcinoma with a massive metastasis in the liver, which is the cause of his current complaints. I've recommended CDE [Cyclophosphamide Doxorubicine Etopiside].'

. . .

He's in bad shape. Very bad. We have to act immediately, otherwise it'll be too late.'

. . .

'The side effects aren't too bad these days. And small-cell lung carcinoma responds well to CDE. It's palliative, and in most cases life-extending. We need to start immediately, and then wait and see.

. . .

'Yes, both he and his wife agreed.'

. . .

'Okay, goodbye.'

'GP?' I ask after he has hung up.

'Yes. He didn't agree with the decision to treat Mr Heuvel with chemotherapy, and of course there is a certain risk in doing it. But if we don't then he's going to die in the very short term. Now at least he has a chance.'

'Does it happen often that GPs disagree with the decision to treat?'

'Yes, sometimes. Some GPs have very outdated ideas about chemotherapy. We try to keep them informed but we don't reach all of them. These days chemotherapy is not as bad for the patient as it used to be.'

Fifteen minutes later the outpatient clinic closes and I rush to the ward to see how Mr Heuvel is getting on. He has been put in a room with five other patients and is being taken care of by one of the nurses, Nanet Jonker. Mrs Heuvel is crying and repeating the story about her husband's appetite. Nanet tries to calm her with a cup of coffee.

'You will need to go home and bring some things for your husband,' she says, giving Mrs Heuvel a list of requirements.

'Toothbrush, pyjamas, razor . . .' Mrs Heuvel repeats the list mechanically.

'And he has a phone next to the bed so you can call,' Nanet adds.

Mrs Heuvel shakes her head. 'He's not one for telephones,' she says.

'Well, if you want to know how he's doing you can always call us,' Nanet says.

Shortly after I meet the doctor in charge of the ward, Frank Terpstra. He informs me that Mr Heuvel will be getting his first course of chemotherapy the same afternoon. He shakes his head and says that Mr Heuvel is really too ill to be sharing a room. He would like to transfer him to a private room.

'I don't think this is going to work,' he says. 'I think he is going to die very soon.' Half an hour later I go to my office to work out my notes. Through the window I see Mrs Heuvel heading toward the bus stop carrying her outsize handbag. She looks forlorn.

Choosing chemotherapy

Mr Heuvel is an example of diagnosis in an already terminally ill patient. It also illustrates the aggressive, explosive growth of small-cell lung carcinoma. Mr Wiersema, who felt quite well at the time of diagnosis, would progress to the same stage as Mr Heuvel in a few weeks. This makes clear why doctors are keen to start treatment as soon as possible. It's not so much that they do not give the patient much time to consider, as there not being much time to consider.

The leading way in which Dr Liem conducted the bad news interview with Mr Heuvel is understandable. Mr Heuvel was too ill to think clearly about his situation, and Mrs Heuvel was too upset.[8] She is unable to distinguish relevant from irrelevant issues. Everything, from the salads to her husband's imminent chemotherapy, appear to be of equal importance. She knows that her husband is seriously ill, but at the same time doesn't seem to realize that he is dying. She puts all her faith in the doctor. When both patient and partner are unable to make decisions then the doctor must do this for them.

How does this apply to the other patients? Both Mr Wiersema and Mr Dekker immediately accepted chemotherapy, insisting that they did not need time to consider the options. They both felt that they did not have a

---

8 Frank (1995) refers to reactions like those of Mrs Heuvel as a 'chaos narrative'.

real choice. Mr Wiersema said he had no option but to take what was on offer, and Mr Dekker spoke of standing with his back against the wall. All the patients in this study said similar things, and this appears to be a more general phenomenon. In another study a patient said, 'when you say I have a choice, you don't realize what it is you're really saying. What you're really doing is putting me up against the wall where I have to wait for the bullet to come' (see Wagener 1987). 'Doing nothing' is not seen as an option, so the choice is a spurious one. In practice both doctor and patient want only one thing: immediate treatment.

2 Doctors and nurses

Small-cell lung carcinoma and treatment

'The patient with small-cell lung carcinoma is often an older male,' Dr Liem says, describing his patient population. Dr Liem is one of the lung specialists in the Ruysdael Clinic who has specialized in lung cancer. 'Although I must admit that there has been an increase in the number of women I've been seeing in the past few years. That's because more women are smoking these days.'

It is late afternoon and we have come to Dr Liem's outpatient surgery where we can talk undisturbed. He normally shares the clinic with two other doctors, but at this time of day it is deserted. Guido Liem chooses his words carefully, as is his habit, except now more so due to the tape recorder on the table between us.

'It starts with a cough, sometimes weight loss, and it looks like an infection. The patient goes to his GP and gets an antibiotic. That doesn't help and sooner or later he's referred to hospital for an X-ray. That's when the ball starts to roll. The patient is referred to a specialist, usually a lung specialist. He comes to the general lung outpatient clinic first. Usually they do a bronchoscopy as well to see exactly what kind of lesion it is, whether it's really an infection. Is it pneumonia for example? Or is it something malignant? In the latter case it's important to identify exactly what kind of malignancy. If it's a small-cell lung carcinoma then we need to find out whether the tumour is limited to the chest or whether it has spread elsewhere. That's important for determining optimal therapy.

'We never operate on patients with small-cell lung carcinoma because at the time of diagnosis it has almost always already spread. We assume from the start that it's a systemic disease. If we know that the tumour is going to recur anyway then we don't like to burden the patient with operations. The metastases aren't always visible on the X-rays and scans because they're usually too small, but we know from experience that they're almost always there.

'We treat all cases of small-cell lung carcinoma with chemotherapy. Unless the patient refuses, of course,' Dr Liem adds quickly. 'Some patients also receive radiotherapy. They're the ones with limited tumour growth; we call that limited disease. As a result of chemotherapy they have a so-called complete remission, which means that all signs of the tumour have disappeared. We then focus the radiotherapy on the spot where the original tumour was. The combination of chemo and radiotherapy gives the optimal chance of becoming a long-term survivor, which means that the patient lives for longer than five years after diagnosis. In the group of limited disease patients that is 8–10 per cent. In the case of some of the newer treatment regimens that we are researching at the moment it's a bit higher, about 15 per cent.

'It's possible that a long-term survivor might be cured, but if you look at the statistics then they still have a higher chance of getting a second malignancy than the normal population. They have a number of cumulative genetic defects and sooner or later these cause derailment of cell growth, which leads to cancer. It's something you have or you don't have.

'Patients with a so-called extended disease – which means that the tumour has extended outside the thorax half in which it originated – are almost all dead within two years. So for the prognosis it's important to know exactly how far the tumour has developed. Because if you know that cure is a possibility then you need to treat as quickly and as intensively as possible. Even if you only cure a small percentage of the patients, you can't afford to lose time. The rate of growth of small-cell lung carcinoma is phenomenal, explosive.

'In the case of those for whom you know that cure is not a possibility the treatment is meant to be palliative. That means that you want to make sure that the tumour causes the patient as little discomfort as possible. The treatment is aimed at improving the patient's quality of life.'

'Is extension of life also part of palliation?' I ask.

'No. Strictly speaking palliation means that you try and alleviate or remove the symptoms, although in practice the lives of this category of patients are also extended. The result of chemotherapy in both limited and extended disease is extension of life, but of course that extension is shorter for patients with extended disease. If you don't treat patients with small-cell lung carcinoma then about half are dead within three months, and half of those within six weeks. Chemotherapy always gives an extension, and we are trying to increase that extension with new treatments. We're doing research with pacletaxel at the moment, for example. There is reliable evidence that we can increase the disease-free interval for patients with small-cell lung carcinoma. When they have completed treatment, patients are okay for a while, but sooner or later the tumour returns. We're trying to extend that tumour-free interval, trying to make small-cell lung car- cinoma a chronic disease. We want to give people who used to die of a dramatic, acute disease within 6–12 weeks a few extra years of life. We do that by treating at large intervals. We treat the tumour, bide our time while it grows, then treat again. You need to realize, though, that it becomes increasingly difficult to treat because the tumour becomes resistant. That means that at a certain point the treatment only works if you have the means of tackling the cell at different points, where it can't develop resistance. You can't go on doing that indefinitely, though, because those cells are clever and they become so resistant that nothing works. That's the end of the road. We have to say to the patient: It's not working any more, we have to stop.

'In the past all patients from this area with small-cell lung carcinoma were treated in this hospital. In that way a whole group of lung specialists were trained in the use of the standard CDE chemotherapy regimen. As a result we no longer get all the patients from the periphery. And that's how it should be. As an academic teaching hospital it's our job to perfect existing therapy and develop new cures and then pass these on to doctors working in the periphery. We teach young doctors new techniques and in that way they spread. Take CDE; it's now standard practice. That wasn't always the case. Ten, 15 years ago nobody used it. We have to focus on the most important medical problems and, as I said, we're now trying to extend the disease-free interval in patients with small-cell lung carcinoma.'

Choosing therapy

'For the patient with small-cell lung carcinoma, once the diagnosis has been made, the question inevitably arises, "How long do I have to live if I don't accept treatment?" The answer to that question is so dramatic, especially for those who do not even feel ill, that they claim they do not have any real choice. I agree with them. With that sort of prognosis, doing nothing is not an option. Dying is not an option that a person can be expected to choose under most conditions. Most patients are still too attached to life to choose death. Part of the reason for this is that the diagnosis takes them by surprise. It's not something that develops gradually. All of a sudden the tumour is there, and at that moment they realize that there are still a lot of things they want to do, a lot of unfinished business. They are not ready to die. So most of them accept chemotherapy immediately. It's the obvious choice.'

'Is it the patient or the doctor who decides?' I ask.

'The doctor usually says, "You have small-cell lung carcinoma and we have to treat it with chemotherapy." For some diseases there are treatments that are so much better than doing nothing. So, yes, I think it's the doctor who decides. And to be quite honest – and this is not a popular opinion – I think that the doctor *has to* decide. But there are, of course, limits.'

'Why do you think the doctor *has to* decide?'

'Because most people just don't have a good enough picture of what the options are. In a situation like that, dominated by desperation and emotion, patients are just not capable of systematically weighing all the options. *That's why they leave the decision to the doctor. They say, "You tell me what's best doctor."* So the doctor has a responsibility, and you have to offer them something that will help. And I think that in the case of patients with small-cell lung carcinoma that is chemotherapy.'

'So why do patients put their lives in the doctor's hands?'

'I think it's primarily a question of trusting the doctor's medical knowledge and expertise. Then secondly, for some people it's not so much the doctor's professional knowledge but his aura. Thirdly, some patients have already consulted other doctors, often quacks, who end up not doing very much. Then they hear about us and when they come they grab everything we have to offer. They want *something* to be done; it doesn't matter what. They don't want to be just left to die.' Dr Liem falls silent.

'So you're happy make the decision for patients because you think that the treatment is beneficial,' I try to summarize.

'Yes,' he nods. 'Of course, I always try to involve them in the decision. I tell them, especially those who are incurable, that they are the only ones who can properly weigh the advantages and disadvantages of treatment. My criterion is whether or not I would do it myself. It's a bit tricky though. I read a study in one of the medical journals. They asked doctors who often have to deal with situations like that what they would do themselves, then it turns out they would be very reluctant to undergo that kind of treatment. Patients, on the other hand, are keen to undergo treatment.' Guido Liem looks at me over the edge of his reading glasses. 'Various other people, relatives, also intervene. And when you look at the kind of treatment that is recommended then that also varies from one doctor to another. So when you present the options to people who are healthy they tend to have objections. It's when they're *sick* that things change. Interviews with doctors who have contracted the disease themselves have shown that from the moment of diagnosis they behave the same as other patients. So when you think abstractly about that kind of decision, you tend to be more conservative about treatment.

'Very occasionally a patient will refuse treatment, but it doesn't happen often. The odd patient refuses because he thinks that he has lived life to the full and his time has come. I can understand that, and if they've thought it through then I respect their decision.' Dr Liem falls silent. 'Problem is,' he continues after a while, 'you're never quite sure whether they have a psychiatric problem. It's something I've been confronted with. Maybe they're depressive. And they do often have a depressive tendency. But usually they're people who have thought deeply about life and death and made a carefully considered decision. I think it's good for that category of patients to say "no", but the large majority, with their background firmly in Dutch culture and values, automatically says "yes" to life.'

'Legal and ethical tracts about patient autonomy talk about patients having to decide themselves,' I say. 'Is that something you see in practice?'

'Only in a small intellectual minority. My patients don't generally belong to that group. I think you have to address patients on their level; sometimes you need to use metaphors to explain. With intellectual patients you can simply present the facts and let them decide for themselves. That's also difficult of course. It doesn't only apply to medical decisions. If you have a financial problem you also get an expert to explain things. If you're not familiar with the subject you can read the literature, inform yourself and then come to a decision. But usually you base your decision on the information and advice provided by an expert.'

'You say that patients with small-cell lung carcinoma are a special category. Is the decision process different for patients with other kinds of cancer? If there were a kind of cancer that affected mainly intellectuals, would they decide more independently, more rationally?'

'Take Mr Post for example,' Dr Liem says. 'Professor of econometrics; someone who could easily distinguish the important from the unimportant. But even in those cases, emotional factors play a role. Mr Post refused treatment, saying he'd rather die, but then a few days later decided to accept treatment after all.'

'Are you saying that he had thought more about his decision than the other patients?'

'Yes,' Dr Liem nods. 'I had the impression that he'd thought about it very seriously. He'd discussed it with his wife and doctor friends. But of course he had feelings about it as well. And they were initially conflicting. It's part of the process of coping. I can imagine that as he talked to various people he gradually adopted their idea that he should accept treatment. But Mr Post also didn't have small-cell lung carcinoma. He had plenty of time to go home for two weeks and think things over. Patients with small-cell lung carcinoma don't have that kind of time. They have to decide immediately otherwise it's too late. It takes them by surprise. But coming back to your question, I think the patient's role in the decision is limited.'

'There's a lot of talk about informed consent and in discussions about ethics we talk about respecting the patient's autonomy. How does that work in practice?'

'I'm familiar with that discussion,' Dr Liem says. 'And to be honest I think it's a lot of rubbish. It's very fashionable these days. I think it's good that these issues are discussed, but sometimes it goes a bit far. You sometimes see professors of ethics discussing chemotherapy on the television, but it's obvious from the start that they have no idea what they're talking about. It's embarrassing, like listening to the Pope talk about contraception. Then I think to myself: why don't you come and spend three months in a hospital so you can see what things are really like. When you're seriously ill you have less time for rational comparisons and highbrow theoretical discussions. You're not interested in those issues, you just want to be emotionally indulged. So when you talk about patient autonomy and the patient having the right to decide . . .' He shrugs. 'I don't think there is any such thing as patient autonomy, or rather, I don't think they have that much autonomy, especially not those who are seriously ill. The sicker you are the less important autonomy is to you. In that phase you deal with things more emotionally, you want emotional attention from loved ones, not to be bothered with the pros and cons of abstract choices.'

Under the spell of *The Riddle*[1]

The narratives of Mr Dekker and Dr Liem are completely different in tone and content, and yet they are both about small-cell lung carcinoma. For the patient the disease is unique, it threatens his very existence. Mr Dekker talks about what the disease means for him and his loved ones, he speaks from his emotions (see Gelauff and Manschot 1997: 195). When Dr Liem hears Mr Dekker's personal narrative of suffering, disease and need he translates it into his own medical discourse, as a physical problem that requires a solution. Dr Liem describes how he listens to the patient's story and extracts those elements that are important for him. He distils a pattern of complaints and symptoms from the narrative. He then organizes the necessary tests in order to come to a diagnosis and confirm his suspicions. Then, finally, he decides on the therapeutic options. He finds the other issues, such as what the illness means for the patient, understandable and unpleasant for the patient but for himself as doctor they are less relevant. These are issues for the relatives, other care providers and psycho-social support staff to deal with. Doctors who are confronted with seriously ill patients have to solve *The Riddle*, they have to make a diagnosis, decide on treatment options and apply them (Gelauff and Manschot 1997: 193).

To put it rather simplistically, for doctors small-cell lung carcinoma is much more a question of a diagnosis that must be made and a disease that needs to be treated than it is for patients. And for specialists in an academic hospital it is also a scientific challenge (which does not necessarily mean that doctors in peripheral hospitals do not have scientific ambitions). The exaggeration here is intentional. Disease (obviously) has different meanings for doctors and patients, and of course doctors do care about patients as individuals and find the human aspects of disease important. But I also want to emphasize the differences between doctors' perspective and the other central perspectives in this book, those of the patients and the nurses.

Unlike the doctors and nurses, I was a temporary participant in the hospital. When I asked doctors how they persevered in a profession in which they were confronted with dying patients week after week, year after year, the answer was that they were not just doctors treating terminally ill patients but also scientific researchers. As Dr Liem put it, 'Doctors in an academic setting should focus on the major medical issues of the moment.' When this has been 'solved' they should move on to the next problem.

The biggest challenge for the academic doctor is not always in the first instance the welfare of individual patients but that of the whole category of patients in general through solving *The Riddle* of the disease.[1] The satisfaction of solving *The Riddle* is a reward in itself and the fuel that drives the clinical motors of the greatest medical specialists; it is the most important aspect of their professional self-image. Of course doctors try to treat their patients with empathy and reduce their suffering. But that is not sufficient to keep them abreast of developments in the field, or even sufficient to maintain their enthusiasm. Even the most dedicated clinicians are driven by *The Riddle*.[2]

Which brings us to the question of academic doctors' double role as clinicians *and* researchers. These are conflicting roles. For the clinician the interests of the individual patient are central, for the researcher it is the interests of science, though in the future the benefits of science may serve the interests of a whole category of patients (Taylor 1984). Caring for individual patients and the interests of medical science do not always coincide (Uden and van Dam 1986).

Clinical trials

Mr Dekker and Mr Wiersema participated in a so-called phase 3 clinical trial.[3] The most important consequence of this was that they had to spend three days in hospital and that blood samples were often needed for the study. In addition, various tests are carried out before and after the treatment. The standard treatment for small-cell lung carcinoma, CDE chemotherapy, can be given in the outpatient clinic. The hospital ethics committee must approve clinical trials before they can be carried out. Patients have to give written informed consent. The procedure entails the doctor giving a brief description of the study (practical details, possible side effects), the

---

1 The term *The Riddle* is taken from Nuland (1995). I define the term slightly differently. He reserves the term for the search for diagnosis. In the case of small-cell lung carcinoma it was usually not a problem to make a diagnosis. The challenge here was more the scientific one of finding a better therapeutic 'solution'. I use *The Riddle* to refer to this latter challenge. The upper case is to emphasize that all other challenges pale in comparison.

2 This paragraph is taken almost literally from Nuland (1995: 261).

3 In phase 1 trials substances that have been shown to have a limiting effect on cell division in a laboratory setting are tried out for safety in a clinical setting. In phase 2 trials these potential new cytostatic drugs are tested for efficacy. Phase 3 trials entail comparing two groups of patients, with one group receiving the current standard treatment and the other group receiving the new drug.

patient receiving and reading an information brochure and then signing a consent form. Just like Mr Dekker and Mr Wiersema, the other patients who were included in the trial hardly asked any questions about the study. They all agreed almost immediately.

The doctors did not go to great lengths to explain the exact nature of the therapy to patients, especially in the choice between the standard treatment and the trial medication in phase 3 trials, as we have seen in the case of Mr Dekker and Mr Wiersema. When they wanted patients to participate in phase 1 and phase 2 trials, doctors were much more explicit about the research nature of the treatment. They defended their limited explanation of phase 3 trials by saying that it was not harmful and was at least as effective as the standard treatment and the patients could read all about it in the brochure. This is true, but one wonders how much they understood of what they read. The consent form is supposed to support the patient. However, handing out forms does not mean that patients read them or understand them (Casselith et al. 1980). When doctors requested written informed consent from patients they supported this by saying, 'It's to make sure I've told you what it's all about,' as though getting informed consent was primarily to protect the doctor against legal action. It is hardly surprising that the patients interpreted it in this way as well (Bolt 1991).

Intermezzo: doctor and anthropologist

Above I have discussed the doctors' medical-technical and scientific perspective. For an outsider this might initially seem difficult to understand; it is easier to identify with the patient. After all, are we not potential patients as well? I experienced this myself during one of the first consultations, in which the doctor was discussing therapy options with a 33-year-old patient and his wife. A week earlier the doctor had told the patient that he was incurably ill. The patient had asked how long he still had and the doctor had replied one or two years. The patient talked about his 6-year-old daughter, asked about the possibility of lung transplantation, and then grasped his wife's hand as he insisted that he would do *anything* to get better. I was touched and remained silent after they had left. I had the idea that I should be able to cope with all kinds of situations in the hospital, including ones like this. I followed the doctor, X-rays and case notes under his arm, down the corridor and past the reception desk. Suddenly he turned round. 'Not your average patient,' he said. 'Yes,' I said, thinking we shared the same empathy 'such a *nice* man, and still so *young*. It's terrible . . .' I stopped, seeing that he was looking at me uncomprehendingly. 'Young, yes,' he nodded sympathetically, 'but a combination of squamous cell *and* adenocarcinoma is very unusual,' he continued enthusiastically. 'I can't remember ever seeing a case like it.'

The exception: the patient who refuses treatment

During my study there were three patients who refused first-line chemotherapy. None of them belonged to the group I was studying and could not have been included in my group for that very reason. Two were patients who had professional experience of cancer patients. Mr Boelens was a 55-year-old employee of the Ruysdael Clinic. For 25 years he had pushed patients in their beds between the wards and the rooms where various tests were carried out. His work area included the General Cancer Department. Mr Boelens looked fit; apart from a persistent cough and occasionally a heavy feeling in the chest he had no complaints. Just as in the case of Mr Wiersema, he responded to the diagnosis with disbelief. He came to see Dr Heller three times. He thought they must have made a mistake. It was inconceivable to him that he could feel fine but be terminally ill. His wife said that he went on gruelling trips on his racing bike every afternoon in order to try and feel the tumour in his lungs so that he could believe the diagnosis. But he tried in vain. During consultations he kept enquiring about the possibility of surgery. Dr Heller repeated that when this kind of tumour had spread, the only option was chemotherapy. Each time Mr Boelens rejected this option. He had seen so many patients struggle through the courses of chemotherapy that did not cure them. Long ago he had decided that if it ever happened to him he would refuse chemotherapy. He stuck to that decision when the time came. Dr Heller said he understood his choice but was sorry that he had refused treatment. He asked him to think about it over the weekend.

During the third meeting Mr Boelens's son came along. He had looked up small-cell lung carcinoma in a medical encyclopaedia. He had read that his father was incurably ill, that he did not have long to live and that treatment was palliative and not curative. Dr Heller added some details but could not avoid agreeing with the broad picture. The son was involved in homeopathy. If his father was incurable and the only option was palliation, then he put more trust in homeopathy. Dr Heller repeated that he respected their decision but that he thought it was a pity. I never saw Mr Boelens again.

The 48-year-old Mrs de Groot had a similar background. She had made the tea and coffee in the Cancer Department for years. She had been admitted with shortage of breath and pain in the chest. When she heard the diagnosis she immediately and persistently refused chemotherapy. She said that she had seen enough of the suffering caused by chemotherapy. A few days later she said that she no longer wanted to live. She felt terrible. She had recently divorced and was bitter about what life had to offer after the fatal diagnosis. The pain increased and she was given morphine. She died two weeks later.

The third patient, Mrs Kassies, had no experience with cancer patients.[4] She suffered from severe COPD (chronic obstructive pulmonary disease), had been rheumatic for years and had had a leg amputated due to some vascular disorder. Because her husband could no longer cope with caring for her at home she had been admitted to a nursing home. There she had become increasingly short of breath. She was referred to hospital where a metastasized small-cell lung carcinoma was diagnosed. Mrs Kassies had suffered pain for years and was at the end of her tether. She had had enough of life. She did not want to be treated if she could not be cured and she did not want any further tests either. After refusing chemotherapy she told one of the nurses that she 'would rather die' and she requested euthanasia. This request caused divisions on the ward. It was not clear whether she really wanted euthanasia or was simply afraid of pain and suffering and troubled by the thought that she had become dispensable. The doctors finally decided that her euthanasia request was 'not genuine' and they did not grant it. She was given morphine for the pain, later in combination with Valium, and she died a week after the diagnosis.

The doctors in question offered these three patients chemotherapy in the same way as they did the patients I was studying. The initiative to refuse treatment came clearly from the patient. The patients' choice was determined to a large extent by aspects of their biographies. In the case of the first two these were their experiences with other cancer patients. Somewhere in the past, quite separate from their own physical condition they had decided that if they were to contract such a disease they would not accept treatment unless it was curative. For Mr Boelens this was crucial. The difference between him and Mrs de Groot was that she gave the impression that she was disappointed with life and that she suffered pain. Mrs Kassies had experienced a long trajectory of personal suffering and did not want to add more. When she heard that she had terminal cancer she decided that that was the end.

I am aware that the patients I saw were a small selection. The patients in the hospital had already passed one gatekeeper: the general practitioner (GP). There are also patients who do not end up in hospital, either through their own initiative or on advice from their GP. Some patients came from peripheral hospitals, though they usually came for second- and third-line chemotherapy and hardly ever for first-line therapy. Those who came from peripheral hospitals had a strong desire for treatment. It is striking that Dr Liem mentioned 'the intellectual patient' several times. The three patients who did refuse therapy did not have a higher education but had thought about life and death, and in this sense could be considered 'intellectual'.

---

4 This patient is discussed in The (1997a: 42–56).

Socio-demographic factors also seem to be relevant. There is a correlation between age and level of education and the desire to participate in the decision-making process. Those with a higher education and those in the younger age groups have a greater desire to participate (Regt et al. 1998: 30). Very occasionally there was a highly educated patient in the clinic. In such cases the communication between doctor and patient was different. There was interaction and the doctor offered more information voluntarily (see Street 1991). These patients also asked many more questions, which led to the doctor giving even more information. Doctors adjust themselves to the patient's 'questioning behaviour'. I had the impression that doctors liked talking to this category of patients because they shared the same social and cultural codes and forms of communication. Doctors appeared to be most receptive to a direct, almost business-like style of conversation with few expressions of emotion. This preference is understandable, as it is a rational and objective conversational style that fits well with the way in which they are used to communicate (The 1997a: 65–6).

The oncology nurse

'The unusual thing about patients with small-cell lung carcinoma is that they come back with clock-work regularity,' Mark van Rossum, oncology outpatient nurse, says. 'The standard CDE therapy consists of three treatments in a week. So for one course of treatment we see them three times. We develop a relationship of trust that becomes more intensive the longer patients and their relatives come to the clinic. The other day I had a lung cancer patient on my list for chemotherapy and I couldn't visualize his face. That's something that almost never happens.

'Nurses who do the rounds have more opportunity to talk to patients. "Doing the rounds" means giving them back their appointment card and perhaps giving further explanation about test results. It's not much. The assistant could also do it, but here the nurses should do it. It doesn't really add anything, except, well, when they've just heard the bad news and they come into the waiting room all upset, then the nurses know what to do. We try to help patients like that as much as possible.

'Of course, there are some patients with whom you don't have that kind of contact. It all depends on the person and the opportunity. If you have the chance to sit with someone and there is no one else around then the conversation is different, you go deeper. When I'm alone with patients I try to use those moments for things like that. Sometimes I say, "If you feel like talking then we can go somewhere where it's quiet."

'Unfortunately the doctors often don't warn us when they are going to give the patient the bad news. If we were present during that first interview then we would know exactly what they had told the patient. But even later, when we know the patient better, it's still a pity that we don't know when they are going to be given bad news. But we keep an eye open. I see them coming out of the doctor's office and it's obvious what has happened. You can see on their faces that they've received bad news. Those are the moments that we try to help them. Sometimes they come to us. They just have to talk to someone. They say they're happy to see someone they know. There seems to be a need for something like that.

'Guido Liem and Ronald Veerman in particular forget to keep us informed. It's a pity, and to tell you the truth it makes me rather angry. It's really inadequate behaviour on their part. It's so much better for patients when we are aware of what's going on and can expand on what's been said. Marcel Heller does keep us informed. He says, "I've just had a bad news interview with so-and-so. Can you have a word with him?" We really value that.

'Generally we come into contact with small-cell lung carcinoma patients unexpectedly. If there is a place then they can be treated immediately. Usually a new patient arrives at the outpatient clinic and the doctor calls us and says, "I've got someone here with a small-cell lung carcinoma who needs chemo urgently, today if possible." And before you know it you have the person in front of you waiting for treatment. Then you have to wait and see what happens. I know what's wrong with them from the kind of treatment they're getting, but I don't know what they know. That's the main problem. I often have the impression that they think, "Come on, give me the treatment then I can go home". Then I wonder whether they really know how sick they are.

'The first encounter is unexpected, for us and for them, and that provides an opening for conversation. I ask them, "Hey, did you know you were going to be coming in for chemotherapy today?" Usually they didn't. Those are the sort of things we need to take into account. Patients are completely overwhelmed by what's happening. I try to get the conversation going, but without forcing things. Usually that's relatively easy. Before they end up in the hospital they have usually already experienced quite a lot, and they tell us about that part of the trajectory spontaneously. In those early conversations I try to get some impression of the situation at home. Do they have a family or relatives who will be able to help later when things get difficult?

'Almost all patients with a small-cell lung carcinoma accept chemotherapy. They say that they have no choice. But of course they *do* have a choice: they can refuse therapy or stop once they've started. If you realize that it isn't improving your quality of life, that it is much worse than you anticipated, then you can always stop. I think most of the patients don't realize that they actually do have a choice, and they hardly ever stop. Sometimes I also have the impression that they continue because they don't want to disappoint the doctor. They want to please him by doing what he thinks is best. If I think that's what's happening I say to them, "If you think it's too much then you must say so."'

'The whole family suffers'

'I often notice that the partners have a harder time with the illness than the patients themselves. I try to notice things like that. Sometimes we have to devote more effort to the partner than to the patient. But that's all part of the job. I see my job as helping the whole family. The patient is the one with the disease but it's really the whole family that is sick, the whole family suffers. The partners themselves tend to forget that. A lot is expected of the partners of patients. Everyone gives them friendly advice. Doctors often say to a spouse, "You should try this or you need to do that," and if it doesn't work then it's really frustrating for them. They have their hands full at home. Usually they have no experience of taking care of the sick, so they have difficulty judging the seriousness of the situation, and that can make them rather hopeless. I think it's particularly import-ant for partners that they get recognition, that we let them know that they are dealing with a very difficult situation and that we are aware of it. The wife of a patient mentioned this to us recently. She said she loved coming to see us because she can talk to us and discuss things, and we understand what caring for her husband entails.

'Talking to patients you'd think there was nothing wrong with them, but when you talk to the partners you find out they're so sick they can hardly get up out of the chair. I think it's because they come from a background in which com-plaining isn't acceptable. But it's also related to the category of patients: usually a bit older, with a tremendous respect for the doctor.

'Listen, if my contact with patients remains on the level of discussing treatment and side effects then it isn't very challenging for me. I think it's important to go further, find out how they are coping more generally, whether the care at home is adequate, whether the partner is able to cope. The interesting thing about my work is to try and piece together all the information to get a more complete picture. Patients tell you the medical part of the story, they tell you the test results were okay. But sometimes I can see that things are not okay, and if I persevere in my questioning then I get very clear answers. And when I combine that information with what the partner has told me I find out that there's a lot more going on than was apparent. Sometimes I also try to influence things, for ex-ample if I think they aren't managing at home and need assistance. If necessary I even call one of the doctors. They're just simple things we can do for them, but they're grateful.'

The nurses' perspective

The last person involved in the treatment of patients with small-cell lung carcinoma whose perspective I want to discuss is the nurse. Elsewhere in this book I discuss the nurses' perspective in detail. Here I want to anticipate that discussion by presenting a brief outline.

Earlier I presented an exaggerated picture of the doctors' primary interest in the patient-as-physical-phenomenon (the symptoms), in the metastasized small-cell lung carcinoma (the diagnosis) and in the therapy as scientific challenge (the clinical trial). The nurse, Mark van Rossum, represents the nurses' perspective. In contrast to the doctors, the nurses are more concerned with the social and emotional aspects of the illness rather than the medical-technical aspects of the disease. They are more interested in the patient as person (Zussman 1992: 64). This is not only a consequence of personal interest but also of the division of labour.

Nurses have a better ear than doctors for the experiential narratives of patients and their partners. They 'follow' the patient's narrative more closely and are less likely to transform the patient's message by giving it medical significance; they are less likely to make a distinction between what is (medically) relevant and irrelevant. Patients are aware that *their* narrative recedes into the background in the doctors' interpretation. This is one of the important reasons for the difference between doctor–patient and nurse–patient interaction (Gelauff and Manschot 1997: 191–3).

When I asked nurses what motivated them to work with terminally ill patients they always said psychosocial support. Mark van Rossum, for example, mentions 'checking whether patients and their family are coping physically and mentally' as one of the challenges of his job. Nurses feel that the patient's social environment, especially the involvement of the partner, also fall under their care. Mark van Rossum refuses to close his ears to the 'complaining' of partners like Mrs Heuvel.

Doctors and nurses have different perspectives on the patient. This is because they are confronted with patients in different ways, they see patients differently and their contact with patients is different. You could say that nurses know the patients and their families better. There is less of a barrier between nurses and patients than there is between doctors and patients. Because the social distance is narrower (differences in education and socialization are smaller) patients and their relatives are often more inclined to raise issues with nurses than they would with doctors. But social class is not the only determining factor here. It is the doctors who make the clinical decisions and who bear the responsibility, not the nurses. Complaints to the doctor about the side effects of treatment can have much wider consequences than the same complaint to a nurse. Patients are dependent (and they feel dependent) on doctors for treatment. In that respect the relationship is asymmetrical (Gelauff and Manschot 1997: 188).

Mark van Rossum mentions this power relationship between doctor and patient. He sees the patients' loyalty toward the doctor, their desire to comply and in particular not to be troublesome. I agree with him in this. The paucity of complaints about the long waiting time in the outpatient clinic and the constant interruptions of the consultation by the doctor's pager struck me. I was also surprised by patients' willingness to undergo all kinds of tests. It seemed as though they were grateful that the doctor was willing to grant them a few moments of his valuable time.

The contact between nurses and patients is also different because nurses are often present at the very moment that patients are having a hard time. Mark van Rossum has to give chemotherapy to patients who have just been diagnosed with lung cancer. Later on as well, when patients learn they have a recurrence, or that the hospital can do nothing more for them, there is usually a nurse in the neighbourhood. But nurses also regularly discuss worries with patients and their partners during the less stressful moments of their illness trajectory.

Another factor is the much longer time that nurses and patients spend together. This is particularly true of the nurses who work on the wards. They help patients with intimate things such as washing, dressing and going to the toilet. When the visitors have gone home and patients lie in their beds worrying then nurses are more accessible than doctors. In the out-patient clinic nurses also spend more time with patients than do doctors, for example when the patient is receiving chemotherapy. Another relevant factor is that there is a greater ratio of nurses to patients than there is of doctors.

Judging from what Mark van Rossum says, nurses would prefer to be present during the bad news interview, as happens on the ward. Nurses do not like being confronted by patients when they are not sure what the doctor has told them about their illness and prognosis. During this study I often encountered nurses who were irritated or disappointed because doctors had not informed them about a bad news interview. They interpreted this as meaning that doctors did not consider their contribution to be important. Nurses do think their contribution is important for both patients and their relatives. Patients often agreed with this.

PART II

Therapy, optimism and
perseverance

3 | The rising curve

The treatment is working

[26 February] Three weeks after the start of treatment, Mr and Mrs Wiersema are sitting in Dr Heller's office. The doctor is concentrating on a set of X-rays. He removes another set of X-rays from a large brown envelope and compares the two. The room is silent. Mr and Mrs Wiersema do not move. They seem to be making every effort not to disturb the doctor's concentration. They occasionally exchange tense glances. The click as Dr Heller sticks another X-ray onto the light box on the wall is harsh in the silence.

My thoughts drift to earlier in the morning when I had spoken to Mr and Mrs Wiersema in the waiting room. Mr Wiersema had been very nervous. He had not slept for three nights because of this. As we talked he avoided eye contact. They were both very anxious to hear the results.

There is a loud beep and Dr Heller's pager brings me back to the present. He turns round, picks up the phone, dials a number and sits down behind his desk.

'Marcel Heller,' he says.

. . .

'What's the problem?' he says, as he writes the patient's name on the back of a lab report.

. . .

'Yes, she qualified for the *carboplatin* radiotherapy study.'

. . .

'My surgery is three times a week, on Mondays, Wednesdays and Fridays. She can make an appointment through the outpatient clinic. She could come this Friday.'

. . .

'Okay.' He hangs up and pages through Mr Wiersema's file. 'Sorry for the interruption,' he says. 'We give a lot of advice to lung specialists in peripheral hospitals, so it's important that we're accessible. Mr and Mrs Wiersema nod. Dr Heller looks at Mr Wiersema's lab results, then he leans over a green form and fills in various details. When he has finished he looks up at the Wiersemas, who have been waiting patiently. 'I'm satisfied,' he says. 'The X-rays look good, the tumour is hardly visible.' He points to the large patch of white on the old X-ray and then to the much smaller patch on the more recent X-ray. Mr Wiersema nods, his face straight, as though this is some routine announcement. The joy is clear on Mrs Wiersema's face.

'So this is good news,' Dr Heller continues. 'The treatment is working.'

The outpatient clinic

I often saw Mr and Mrs Wiersema in the outpatient clinic. They would see me scanning the waiting room and Mr Wiersema would put his hand up. As I walked toward them Mrs Wiersema would move up so that I could sit between them. This became a routine. On these occasions Mr Wiersema would never look me in the eye. He was always tense during these visits and he did not sleep well the night before his appointment.

Most patients are nervous before a hospital appointment. This is not too bad during the therapy, but increases when test results are expected. A lot depends on these interviews with the doctor. Patients attach more weight to what the doctors says than to what they feel themselves. If the doctor says everything looks fine and he is satisfied, then all the complaints of a few minutes ago seem to disappear.

The Ruysdael Clinic is an academic centre and so attracts patients from far and wide. Many patients travel for hours to reach the Clinic. In addition to the fact that travelling is tiring in itself, many patients also experience the journey as a source of anxiety. On the way to hospital it is difficult to think of anything other than the illness. Dr Heller once told me that the mere view of the city skyline made some patients nauseous.[1]

---

1 It is not trouble and affliction for all patients, however. Mrs Fisher-Rijn seems to enjoy her visits to the hospital. They are an excursion. The hospital bus that picked her up drove through the villages between her home and the city, stopping on the way to pick up other patients. She chatted on the bus and continued the banter in the waiting room. Not all patients valued this, as her remarks sometimes made them afraid. If a patient was wheeled through the waiting room on a trolley she would nudge her neighbour and say, 'Look, before we know it we'll be like that as well.' During consultation with her favourite doctor, Dr Liem, she would complain about everything, her illness, the treatment and other minor complaints. She would negotiate treatment, 'I'll continue with treatment if you come and visit us at home. I'll make potato salad for you.' When the consultation had finished she updated Dr Liem on the dog shows to which she took her poodles. In the hospital Mrs Fisher-Rijn received the attention that she missed at home. Her husband thought that she exaggerated and that his mild COPD was much worse than her illness. Initially he

Mr Wiersema

[3 March, morning] Mr and Mrs Wiersema are in the visitors' room waiting for laboratory results. The previous week Mr Wiersema's blood had not recovered sufficiently and now he has come for another test. Whether or not he will get another course of treatment depends on the test results. The assumption is that everything will be okay.

'Hey, hello,' Mr Wiersema calls when he sees me. His voice is jolly but his eyes dart about nervously. Every time there is a noise in the corridor he looks nervously at the door. 'I do hope my blood is okay, so I can get my treatment today,' he says. He tells me that he was nauseous during the previous course of treatment, but that he recovered quite quickly.

'I'm going to work on this seriously,' he says.

Mrs Wiersema nods in agreement. 'We have to,' she says.

'I'm not planning to die within six months, you can be sure of that.'

[3 March afternoon] During the course of the day I see Mr Wiersema leave the ward on a number of occasions. When I run into him on the stairs, I ask him where he has been going. He winks conspiratorially and puts a finger to his lips. 'Shhhh,' he whispers. He glances nervously over his shoulder as he takes something from the pocket of his dressing gown. He opens his hand to reveal a matchbox. Still glancing around nervously he slides the matchbox open. It contains a cigarette butt. 'I have to keep nipping up to the smoking room to take a few drags,' he explains. 'Then I pinch off the end and put it back in the matchbox. But the corridors are dangerous; lots of doctors passing by. I regularly see Dr Heller.'

'I thought you'd given up?'

'Yes, it's really bad for you. I'm trying everything. I just take the odd drag. I'm reducing gradually.'

'I think it'll be gone after three courses of treatment'

[31 March] 'Hey, girlie!' I'm pushing the trolley down the corridor collecting dirty cups. 'Hey, girlie!' I hear again, coming from room 102. I let go of the trolley, take two steps backward and peer into the room, straight into Mr Wiersema's laughing face. He is sitting on his bed, his arm connected with various tubes to the infusion standard next to his bed. His hair is becoming thin and wispy.

'Mr Wiersema, hello,' I say, surprised.

'Here I am again,' he says, spreading his arms.

'Yes, I can see that. How are you?'

---

accompanied her and monopolized the doctor's attention for his own complaints. Dr Liem 'dealt' with him by transferring him to the 'ordinary' lung outpatient clinic. With her husband no longer around she seemed a lot happier and attached other activities to her hospital visits, such as lunch in the hospital canteen.

'Fine. Today's the third course.'

I look at the next bed, where Mr Koster, who is participating in the same trial as Mr Wiersema and Mr Dekker, is buried deep beneath his blankets, with only his face visible. He is pale and his eyes are shut tightly. Mr Wiersema looks at his neighbour and shakes his head.

[31 March afternoon] Shortly before the afternoon nursing shift hands over to the evening shift I'm sitting behind the ward reception desk when I see Mr Wiersema, his infusion stand in hand, shuffling toward the door. He waves and winks when he sees me looking.

'Feel like a change of environment?' I ask as I take a seat next to him in the hall.

'Yes, that as well,' he answers. 'I get bored here. But now I had to leave. In the afternoon Mr Koster's daughter comes to wash him, and then I leave the room. He's too ill to wash himself and he doesn't want the nurses to do it for him. He's having a hard time with the treatment, and it makes him nauseous. Last time I shared a room with Dekker. I get on well with him. We've got . . . how shall I put it? We've got a lot in common. Same disease, same stage in the treatment regimen, same attitude. You get talking, and that's nice. You keep running into each other. We always sit together in the waiting room. He should have been here today, but I haven't seen him yet. Maybe his blood hasn't recovered.'

'Mr Koster also has the same illness, doesn't he?' I ask.

'Yes, but he's a course further, just like Bokjes in the next room. But they're different to Dekker. I prefer Dekker.

'So how are you feeling now?' I ask.

'Good,' he says. 'I had a check-up yesterday. Dr Liem was very happy with the new X-rays.' Mr Wiersema presses his lips together and nods seriously. 'Very good,' he emphasizes. I think I'm lucky that I started so early. When Koster started, his tumour was as big as a fist. Mine was like a matchbox, with a few spots in the liver. Nothing more. After one course of treatment the spots had disappeared and the tumour in the lung was hardly visible. All that's left in the lungs is a trace, nothing worth mentioning according to Dr Liem. I saw it myself on the X-ray. I think that *it* will have completely disappeared after three courses,' Mr Wiersema says meaningfully. The final two courses won't really be necessary. They're just an extra.'

'Extra?'

'Just in case, I mean,' Mr Wiersema says.

Mr Wiersema's secret

[1 April, morning] I give up the chance to have coffee with the nurses so that I can join Mr Wiersema for coffee in the hall behind the large potted plants.

'Does your work bring you to all parts of the hospital?' he asks when we are seated.

'Lung ward' I answer. 'The wards are different to the outpatient clinic, so I have to include both.'

'You're particularly interested in *my* illness, aren't you?'

'Yes, your illness in particular. How you experience it, how your wife experiences it, how you discuss it with the doctor.' I go through my usual introductory talk. Mr Wiersema appears not to be listening.

'I must tell you something,' he says impatiently, interrupting my presentation. 'It's something that might be very important for your research,' he continues, conspiratorially. I look at him questioningly. 'No,' he says, 'perhaps this isn't the time to tell you.'

'Then perhaps you'd better not,' I say. He falls silent and I try to change the subject.

'Okay, okay,' he says, 'I suppose I'd better tell you.' He leans forward and I reciprocate by moving my chair a bit closer.

'I'm doing something else, outside the hospital,' he whispers. When he sees I haven't understood he explains further. 'Chemotherapy is not the only thing I'm taking. That's why things are going so well. But Dr Liem and Dr Heller mustn't find out.'

'Oh, what are you taking?'

'Listen, I'm not interested in nonsense, but just before they gave me the final diagnosis my neighbour said that he knew someone who could help. He told me that his colleague's daughter had been terminally ill, and the hospital they had given up hope. The colleague tried everything and nothing worked. Then finally he heard about Natasha. You won't believe it, but a year later the daughter was cured. She's better! My neighbour said, "Natasha's a very busy woman, but she'll see you if I put in a word." And it's not expensive, so what have I got to lose?

'I went to see Natasha on the Friday, just before they told me definitively on the Monday that I had cancer. She told me, "Joop, things look bad. You've got a tumour, and it's wrapped around an artery. That tumour's strangling you." And what do you think they told me on the Monday? Exactly! That they couldn't operate because the tumour was connected to an artery.' Mr Wiersema looks at me triumphantly. 'That's when I knew that Natasha was the right person to treat me.'

'But what does she do exactly?' I ask.

'She's a hypno-therapist. Listen, the idea is that we're not here for the first time. This isn't our first life. We're continually being reincarnated. Things that happened in a previous life influence this life. Long ago I must have experienced something that's still bothering me. In the sixteenth century I went to war as a 14-year-old boy. I was stabbed and died of my wounds. I've still got that wound, and guess where it is.' He points to his chest. 'Exactly here. Natasha says I have to work through that experience, and to do that I have to go back to my past. And as long as I don't deal with it I'll continue to die from problems in my lungs in each new life. Cancer is the war of our time. That's how it is. If I succeed in dealing with my problem then I'll be cured. Natasha says I'm making good progress.'

'But tell me what she does,' I say, curious. 'You arrive and what happens next?'

'Yes, I arrive and then . . . It's in her house, she has a special room. I have to sit on a stool. The room's dark. Natasha is very concentrated, and she hypnotizes me. Then she gets me to talk about my experiences. I don't notice it at the time, but afterwards I'm exhausted. The next day I feel like a new man, like I've been given more space.'

'Unbelievable,' I say.

'You have to have been there to believe it,' Mr Wiersema says. I also thought it was nonsense at first. She's really nice. I go there three times a week. I always carry her phone number with me. I can always call if I'm not feeling well, and then she comes to treat me, even right here in the hospital. I've never done that, but it's good to know that it's possible. My wife also goes to Natasha, for her nerves. This whole situation has made her very tense. If I'm not doing well then she gets nervous.'

'What a story,' I say.

'But it's still a secret,' Mr Wiersema repeats, looking at me strictly.[2] I nod. 'Let me tell you what Natasha said last Tuesday,' he continues. After the session she told me that the tumour had *dried up*, that it had *shrivelled.*' With his hands he shapes a large ball that gradually gets smaller. 'It means that I'm cured. That's why I'm in such high spirits, understand?' He looks at me questioningly. 'Now you understand, don't you?' I nod, somewhat bewildered.

'What do you think?' he asks.

'If that's true then it's wonderful, of course,' I try to choose my words carefully. 'But if it's true, why are you still coming to the hospital? That's not necessary any more, is it?'

'The chemo is more important than Natasha,' he answers decidedly, as though he'd prepared for this question. 'I'm going to finish the chemo whatever happens, Natasha knows that as well.'

Alternative therapies

Of the 30 patients in this study there were eight who made use of alternative therapies. The therapy varied from various kinds of diet, vitamins and homeopathy to hypnotherapy, positive thinking and drinking 'irradiated water'. The proportion using alternative therapies in this study was higher than that reported by van der Zouwe (1994). In her study, of the 9.4 per cent of patients who were currently using alternative therapy, 5.8 per cent had used alternative therapy at some time and 7.9 per cent had considered

---

2 Later he tells everyone about his experiences with Natasha.

its use. Patients with metastasized tumours with a progressive prognosis and receiving palliative treatment might be more likely to seek cure in the alternative sector. The majority of patients who used alternative therapy in my study started immediately after diagnosis. Crisis moments in the illness trajectory – diagnosis, sudden deterioration – were usually the immediate reason for initiating alternative therapy. One patient, however, did visit a faith healer called Jomande before he heard his diagnosis. She called him up onto the stage and warned him of the illness that had not yet been diagnosed.

The one common factor was that all these patients used alternative therapy *in addition to* regular biomedical treatment. They did not seem to experience the combination as problematic and some even thought that the two therapies went well together. If they were given the choice of using only one form of therapy then all patients would, like Mr Wiersema, choose biomedicine.[3]

The hope of cure was, obviously, a motivating factor for patients utilizing alternative therapies. However, my impression was that being able to actively 'do something' was more important. In other words, seeking alternative treatment stemmed from the patients' reluctance to sit around passively and 'do nothing' (Brinkman-Woltjer et al. 1988: 2322). Anything was better than sitting at home, passively waiting for whatever might happen. Patients often 'know' that alternative therapies do not work, but at least they are actively doing something about their illness. It gives them a sense of control.

Patients who used magical forms of therapy, like Mr Wiersema, kept this secret from the doctors, while those who used naturalistic therapies, such as vitamins or diets, tended to be more open. The latter were sometimes concerned that the alternative treatment might interfere with the biomedical therapy.

The use of alternative therapies is also related to dissatisfaction with biomedicine (Sharma 1996: 252). In many respects alternative therapy is the opposite of biomedicine with its scientific theories and hierarchical doctor–patient relationship. Patients told me that they received more personal attention from their alternative healer and that they could discuss things much more extensively. Here van Dantzig's comment, that the desperate quest for salvation stems from inadequate psychosocial support in the biomedical setting, is pertinent (van Dantzig 1993: 21–6). But it also stems from the hopeless nature of the illness. Van der Zouwe thinks that the popularity of alternative cancer therapies will decline once effective forms of treatment have been developed. As long as there is no real cure, cancer will invoke fear. The use of alternative therapy is one way in which patients try to come to terms with this fear (van der Zouwe 1994: 146). According to van Dantzig people always try to find solutions, and when they cannot find clinically proven answers they turn to other sources. When biomedicine

---

3 The preceding two paragraphs are based on van der Zouwe (1994: 146).

runs out of solutions then patients seek hope elsewhere. Van der Zouwe claims that it is not alternative therapy per se that should be discussed with the patient but rather their fears, uncertainties and questions relating to their illness and to biomedical therapy.

Earlier I stated that alternative therapy derives its popularity from its different approach and the way in which the therapist interacts with patients. This is not entirely true, however, because both alternative medicine and biomedicine are part of the same cultural paradigm. What they both have in common is that patients seek help from *others* and assume that only *professional experts* can provide health and happiness (Sharma 1996: 252).

Mr Dekker and Mr Wiersema support each other

[1 April, afternoon] The next day Mr Dekker is admitted for a course of treatment. Mr Wiersema arranges to have himself moved to his friend's room. Whenever I pass I hear them talking loudly and laughing. During visiting hours their room is full of relatives. When I peep round the door Mr Dekker calls, 'Look guys, that's Anne-Mei. She always has time for a chat'. He insists I come in and sit next to his bed. The mood is jolly, almost too jolly.

'They're just like two little boys,' Mrs Dekker says to me. I phoned Klaas this morning to find out how things were and he had the giggles. Couldn't get a serious word out of him and I had to hang up. Apparently Joop Wiersema had put on an apron and was dancing round the room.'

'Ach,' Mrs Wiersema interjected, 'it's better than grumpy faces.'

The following day Mr Dekker has blood samples taken and an infusion needle inserted. He lies on his bed bravely and receives the needles without a complaint. I frown at him and he shrugs nonchalantly. Later his wife comes for a visit. We drink coffee together and she talks about Vera, their adopted daughter, who is applying for a job. Referring to the illness they both say that you should not 'just sit by and do nothing'.

When Mr Dekker leaves the room briefly, Mrs Dekker says that he is having a hard time with his illness. When she arrived he had complained that the needles were becoming too much for him. 'You really need each other in times like this,' she says. 'We cry together for a while and then we can cope again for a while.' When she has gone I sit next to his bed and he tells me that *she* is having a hard time. All the hospital visits, for example. He tells me that when he phoned her the previous evening at half past nine she had already gone to bed. Some of the villagers had started to avoid her and friends who they had supported in difficult times were nowhere to be seen. That was really affecting her.

[3 April] After the weekend the atmosphere had changed completely. Mr Wiersema lay in bed, pale and silent. The chemotherapy had made him very nauseous this time, he tells me. His friend Mr Dekker does not disturb him. At half past nine

Mr Wiersema, wearing a coat and a cap, sits in a chair next to his bed waiting impatiently for his wife. When she arrives she is about to install herself, ready for a chat, but Mr Wiersema is not in the mood. He has had enough of the hospital. He wants to go home, to shower in his own bathroom, and eat home cooking. Before she can sit down he gets up, waves to us, 'Dekker, Anne-Mei, see you next time,' and leads her out of the room.

When they have left Mr Dekker tells me how Mr Wiersema became ever more silent during the weekend. He was nauseous all the time.

'How was your treatment?' I ask.

'Mine was also more difficult than usual,' he admits. 'But I think Wiersema had a harder time than I did. I left him alone. I did a bit of reading and painted my soldiers.'

A period of relative mental calm

During treatment patients become calmer and I refer to this as a period of 'relative mental calm'. The extreme desperation after hearing the bad news and the concomitant existential crisis are no longer dominant. The feelings of sadness are under control and gradually recede into the background. Mr Wiersema and Mr Dekker try to establish a new equilibrium with their loved ones. They succeed in this reasonably well because they can orient themselves to a new future: treatment. Therapy diverts attention from the fatal diagnosis.

They have less time to worry. Patients have to attend the clinic regularly for treatment, check-ups and tests. They have to travel and spend time in waiting rooms.

At home they need time to recover from the therapy. Patients have to 'work' on their illness. It is as though they have been given a part-time job, which they carry out with dedication. Their approach is characterized by a positive attitude, no complaints, and perseverance. Partners are also kept busy, with hospital visits and an increased burden of care at home. Most lung cancer patients are men. Their wives put a lot of effort into preparing meals. They buy special vitamins and expensive cuts of meat, prepare stock. It is all they can do and they do it with devotion.

For both patients and partners it is good when 'something' is happening. Just like Mr Dekker and Mr Wiersema, many patients with small-cell lung carcinoma are hard working people who want to 'do things'. They are not used to being passive. For them nothing could be worse than just sitting around and waiting to see how the disease proliferates. As Dr Liem put it, it is not part of Dutch culture.

The hospital provides structure. One course of therapy follows another. In between there are check-ups, X-rays, scans, blood tests. There is always something to focus on. The short-term perspective is dominant and not much thought is given to the long-term. Treatment and hospital visits divide life up into small manageable sections. Each section successfully completed is an achievement and that reduces the general fear (Frank 1995). Working on treatment means 'doing something' to the frightful disease process. It is also reassuring when the doctor declares that he is satisfied with the way treatment is going. I refer to this part of the illness trajectory as 'calm' because there is a certain mental peace. For a while patients do not need to think of the future. 'Relative' peace because, as I have made clear above, absolute peace is out of the question.

The hospital becomes a familiar environment. Patients learn to find their way around and strange faces become familiar. They meet people and make new friends. Like Mr Wiersema and Mr Dekker, patients seek each other's company. Mr Wiersema and Mr Dekker arranged to share a room when they were in hospital together and they always sat together in the out-patient clinic waiting room. When they were at home they kept in touch by telephone. Their wives also enjoyed talking together. This social interaction made hospital visits more pleasant. But it also gave added support; there was no need to explain everything to a fellow-sufferer and the relationship was equal. The recognition (in both senses) was important. Most patients experience meetings with fellow patients as positive (see Costain Schou 1993: 245). When they are together they can be themselves. The loud laugh-ter and rough humour among some groups of patients were an expression of this. Humour reduces fear and makes it manageable. Patients give in to this need in their interaction with each other because it would not be con-sidered appropriate in other social settings. This is because their illness makes the relationships with family and friends more difficult. They try to protect each other and do not want to make the other worry unnecessarily. Friends and acquaintances often avoid the patient because they find contact with cancer confrontational. They are not sure how to react and it is easier to stay away. Patients and their partners find this social ostracism difficult to cope with. Patients often told me that they did not like venturing out in the neighbourhood to go shopping. They noticed that people fell silent when they approached and it made them ill at ease. One couple told me that they had started going to the hospital hairdresser instead of their usual neighbourhood one because at least in the hospital they were treated as normal.

Sometimes, on the other hand, they received too much attention. Patients and their partners complained about having to endlessly repeat 'how things were'. As one partner put it, 'It's all done with good intent, but it forces you to keep talking about it [the illness].' In addition, it is also difficult to adequately explain to 'outsiders' what they are experiencing. More than once I heard patients complain, 'They don't understand what we're going through.'

4 Rescue therapy

Discussion about Mr Heuvel's treatment

[1 April, afternoon] In the single room next door to Mr Dekker and Mr Wiersema, Mr Heuvel is receiving his first course of chemotherapy. He is having problems with the side effects and, as Dr Liem had predicted, he feels sicker than when he was first admitted. Many of the nurses do not agree with the decision to give him chemotherapy given his poor condition. Everyone agrees that he will not last long.

[7 April] Ward rounds are held twice a week. Prior to that all patients are discussed in detail. The discussion is led by the supervisor and is partly intended as a training exercise for junior doctors. Nurses, medical students and sometimes even social workers and physiotherapists participate.

'Mr Heuvel is a rather strange case,' Dr Frank Terpstra begins. 'He came in on the 1st of March. Born in 1930. In all probability a small-cell lung carcinoma with liver metastases. In the outpatient clinic they suspected a primary tumour in the lungs. The large tumour in the abdomen was the most obvious, though. We decided he had a small-cell lung carcinoma and gave him CDE chemotherapy. He then presented with serious liver function disorder. He received a kind of "rescue chemotherapy" in the sense that we didn't do any further tests. If we had waited for those he would certainly have died. He is tired, nauseous and lacks appetite.'

'He's vomiting congealed blood,' Mira Kuipers says. She is the nurse who looks after Mr Heuvel.

'Yes, that's something new,' Dr Terpstra says. There might be an obstruction. It's really an enormous tumour. It's possible to talk to him, though. He's capable of answering questions clearly. I have the impression that he also has ascites. I wanted to do an ultrasound, but he's too ill for that. I've discussed with the family. It's quite possible that it won't end well.'

'Let's see the X-rays,' Dr Bron, the supervisor, says. Dr Terpstra hangs up the X-rays. 'Mmm, there are all kinds of things here that don't belong here,' Dr Bron says. 'Wonder what it is? Is he still nauseous, Frank?'

'Yes,' Dr Terpstra nods. 'He's not eating at all. The tumour in the abdomen has reduced. I think he has ascites. Leukopenic, especially if he's still vomiting congealed blood. He'll probably need a transfusion.'

'A good response like that does make one think of a small-cell lung carcinoma,' Dr Bron remarks as he looks at the X-rays.

'I'm not sure what else we can do,' Dr Terpstra says and looks questioningly at the supervisor.

'Let's wait and see how he does on therapy,' Dr Bron answers. 'We can't do much else.'

'Yes, then at least we've tried it,' Dr Terpstra says.

'Mr Heuvel says that if he'd known that the treatment would make him so ill then he'd have refused it,' Mira Kuipers says carefully. 'Maybe we should keep that in mind when considering a second course of therapy?'

Dr Bron looks sceptical. 'If the therapy works then it's quite possible that a second course won't affect him as badly.' He shakes his head. 'But perhaps that's being a bit too optimistic.'

'I think so,' Dr Terpstra says. 'He's *really* sick, Diederik.'

'The patient's situation is very important,' Dr Bron says. 'Patients generally cope with CDE therapy reasonably well. In this case it will depend on his general condition.'

During this period there are animated discussions between some of the nurses and Dr Terpstra about the reanimation/resuscitation policy. One nurse thinks that Mr Heuvel should not be resuscitated and that he should not be sent to Intensive Care in case of an emergency. The doctor does not think the time is right for decisions of that kind.

'We've just started treatment,' he says in support of his decision. 'In the case of this patient it's a question of all or nothing. And we've already made the decision to go for it. Resuscitation and Intensive Care are part of that package. If he deteriorates we'll have to re-evaluate the situation. And in any case, I can't sell non-resuscitation to the oncologists. They think that patients on therapy should always be resuscitated.'

Outside in the corridor he complains to me, 'Patients have hardly been admitted to the ward and the nurses are already going on about resuscitation.'

Later the nurse in charge of Mr Heuvel says to me, 'Doctors behave as though asking for some clarity about the policy for a particular patient means that we want them to die. Of course we don't. They forget that we are the ones who have to deal with the patient's heart attack in the first instance. If we don't know what the policy is we have to jump on the patient and apply heart massage. In that situation we can't first go and enquire about the policy. Sometimes that happens and the patient ends up dying in Intensive Care anyway. Then the IC nurses or the doctor complain that we shouldn't have imposed resuscitation on a patient in that condition in the first place. When that happens I feel really guilty. That's why I insist on a clear policy beforehand. Mr Heuvel is so sick, it flies in the face of my intuition to reanimate him. I almost feel that if I saw he was having a heart attack I'd go for a walk around the block.' Then, feeling slightly shocked at her own remark she adds, 'I probably wouldn't, though, really.'

The treatment obsession

Mira Kuipers is one of a group of nurses who do not think that Mr Heuvel should be treated. She hates what she calls the doctors' treatment obsession. Later I ask her what she means.

'I'll give you an example,' she says. 'A while ago Frits Cazemier was admitted to the ward. He was so bad he looked as though he was going to die right here in the corridor. He was still quite young. Apparently he had been at home on his deathbed, with his family all gathered round. Everyone had thought he had lung cancer, but a test revealed that it was probably testicular cancer, something that is curable in theory. Suddenly the doctors changed their policy, he could be cured, so they rushed him to hospital.

'I had to care for him and I found that really difficult. He was in so much pain he could hardly move. With a sort of crane I had to lift him up to weigh him so they could decide on how much medication he needed. Then he had to undergo an unpleasant puncture. This all flew in the face of what I intuitively felt he needed. I complained to colleagues and found that they felt the same way about it. We all agreed that he could not survive chemotherapy. Frits himself thought he was going to die; he *was* dying. And then suddenly they say, "We can cure you". His family then believed that he would recover. They had been given hope and of course they wanted to take the chance. I didn't believe it would work, but obviously I couldn't say that to the family. So we, the nurses, decided we weren't going to take him for the puncture. We had a discussion with the doctors responsible. They insisted he had a chance. They kept saying, "But what if he *does* make it?" They gave examples of similar cases in which patients had left the hospital cured. We thought he would only live for a few hours longer. We had a real problem with the fact that we were depriving him of a peaceful death.

'Anyway, it was good that we all discussed it openly. The doctors persevered with the chemotherapy. I can understand that as well, I suppose, because testicular cancer can be cured. But Frits died four days later very unpleasantly. It would have been better if he had been spared all that suffering in the hospital during his final days and been allowed to die peacefully. Frits really suffered before he was *allowed* to die.

'That's an extreme example of the treatment obsession. Mr Heuvel is a different case; he can't get better, so there's no need to go all the way. He's also going to die in a few days, at most a couple of weeks. And they're also depriving him of a peaceful death. It's terrible.'

'But what else can they do?' I ask.

'The point is that the doctors only emphasize chemotherapy. That's too one-sided. They should discuss all the options with the patient. They should explain the implications of *not* accepting chemotherapy. They should make clear that "doing nothing" is also an option, that "doing nothing" doesn't mean that they abandon you to your fate. Patients often think that if they don't accept chemotherapy then they will suffer a lot of pain or choke to death. They don't realize that there is also *ordinary* palliative care. There are all kinds of ways of making their final days comfortable.'

The nurse who takes over Mira Kuipers's shift has a different opinion. 'Yes,' she says, 'he's very sick and I doubt he'll make it, but I think it was a good decision to treat him. It gives him and his relatives the chance to get used to the idea that he is dying.'

The 'dip' after chemotherapy

[14 April] During visiting hours I talk to Mr and Mrs Heuvel. Mr Heuvel seems to have recovered somewhat and can sit up in bed. They are both looking forward to a visit from their son and daughter-in-law who live in Belgium.

[15 April] The next day I look into Mr Heuvel's room and see a completely different spectacle. The curtain round his bed is drawn and the room is full of people. Mr Heuvel in unconscious and Mrs Heuvel is emotional. When she sees me she grabs my hand and sobs into my T-shirt. 'I can't believe it,' she keeps repeating. 'He was so well yesterday.' Around the bed relatives sit in stunned silence.

[Rounds] 'Next we have Mr Heuvel, a man with small-cell lung carcinoma. We haven't done much in the way of diagnostics because he's in such bad shape,' Frank Terpstra summarizes. We established the diagnosis on the basis of an abdominal puncture: possibly metastasized small-cell lung carcinoma for which he is being treated with CDE. Initially there were a lot of problems: jaundiced, nauseous, leukopenic, transfusion of red cells and thrombocytes. An abdominal ultrasound revealed ascites. The metastases have reduced. There is a red lesion on the left leg. Yesterday his temperature was 39.6°C. Cold shivers . . . somewhat confused . . . antibiotics . . . ' the voice drones on.

'His temperature has gone down to 38.4°C this morning,' Dr Bron reads from a report.

'I couldn't interpret that as an abscess,' Dr Terpstra says. 'There is a lesion, but we need to make sure it doesn't develop further.'

'Do we have more recent X-rays so that we can see if the lung abscess is getting smaller?' Dr Bron asks. He gets up to study the new X-ray. 'It seems as though the treatment is having an effect. But we're basing this entirely on what's happening in the abdomen.'

'I've cancelled the gastroscopy,' Dr Terpstra says. He was septic. Wasn't as nauseous. I think we should feed him parentally.'

'What a situation,' Dr Bron sighs, shaking his head.

'How much shall we give him? A litre?' Dr Terpstra asks as he makes notes in the file. 'I spoke to his family yesterday evening and told them that we'll have to wait and see how things develop. I think that the time has come to agree on a non-resuscitation policy.'

'I agree,' Dr Bron nods, then, shaking his head, 'he's already been here two weeks.'

'What's the prognosis?' one of the medical students asks.

'The average prognosis in a case like this, if you do nothing, is three months. If you do do something it's a bit longer. But in this particular case I think we're talking of weeks rather than months.'

[16 April] Mr Heuvel's family has been at his bedside all night. The antibiotics have had an effect: the fever has subsided. Mrs Heuvel has not had much sleep; every sound had her worrying. By afternoon the small room is again filled with friends and relatives. Mr Heuvel is unconscious. The first thing he said when he awoke, his wife tells me through the tears, is that he was disappointed that he had had no visitors. 'The visitors were here,' she had told him, 'but *you* weren't'.

'Yes,' Mr Heuvel says to me, 'now we'll just have to wait and see what happens.'

On the 23rd of April Mr Heuvel receives his second course of chemotherapy. He agrees to this by telling Dr Terpstra that they should do whatever they thought was best. After all, they had studied these things and he had not. Jacob Korte does not agree with this decision. In the corridor he stops Dr Terpstra. 'Mr Heuvel has just been taken out of the jaws of death. The second course of treatment is often much harder than the first.' He doesn't think Mr Heuvel will survive a second course. 'Is this something we should impose on him in his final few days of "life"?' he asks. Frank Terpstra thinks that now is the time to persevere.

'After all, hadn't the therapy had an effect?' he explains to me later. 'Those nurses can be really difficult sometimes,' he continues. 'When you've reached this point you have to continue. He's already had the worst. His GP phoned, insisted that we shouldn't give him another course. He was opposed to treatment right from the start.'

After completing his course of treatment Mr Heuvel is kept in hospital so that the doctors can keep an eye on him during the post-treatment 'dip'. He is soon up and about and I talk to him frequently. He keeps repeating that he was more dead than alive when he was first admitted. He says that things are getting better. 'Every day is a day extra,' he says. A week later he is able to shower by himself, and is to be discharged after the weekend.

The opposing perspectives of doctors and nurses

I have chosen to describe Mr Heuvel's 'rescue therapy' because it illustrates the different, and often contradictory, perspectives of doctors and nurses. In the case of both Mr Heuvel and Frits Cazemier therapy was the priority. The aim of therapy in the former was life-extension, in the latter it was cure. Both patients would have died in the very short-term without treatment. The doctors argued that the goal justified the means. They considered that, in order to achieve this goal, it was legitimate – even necessary – for the patient to suffer.

Generally speaking, nurses are much less inclined to treat whatever the cost. They tend to focus more on the adverse effects of treatment than on the results. And they are more sceptical as to whether results can be achieved. It often seems as though doctors and nurses anticipate the outcome of treatment differently. But it is not only that they differ in whether or not treatment will have an effect, they also differ in the *value* they attach to the small chance that treatment will work. In the cases of Mr Heuvel and Frits Cazemier both doctors and nurses were sceptical that the patients would survive treatment. But the slim chance of success was, for the doctors, reason enough to persevere with treatment, whereas for the nurses it was a reason not to treat. Cases in which everything possible is done to treat a patient and the patient dies anyway are the ones the nurses remember, whereas the doctors always refer to that one successful case, even though it might have been years ago.

Nurses are generally more conservative and more reluctant when it comes to treating patients who are in very bad shape and whose chance of survival is small. In such cases nurses often appeal for a more humane approach (Zussman 1992). Like Mira Kuipers, nurses often have a problem with the doctors' propensity to treat. Their focus is more on care, quality of life, and counselling (The 1997a: 199).

The value of rescue therapy is often determined retrospectively. If it is successful then the doctor is a hero (Zussman 1992). I often noticed that in cases, like that of Mr Heuvel, in which nurses were critical of the doctors' approach and the patient recovered (temporarily) they then retracted their criticism. Mr Heuvel was a success story, in that he survived for another year and a half. One of the nurses who had looked after him during the rescue therapy ran into him and has wife nine months later. Mr Heuvel looked well and said he had enjoyed the summer. The nurse later said that she was glad she had run into him because she now understood why the doctors always insisted on treating.

However, if the rescue therapy does not work, as in the case of Frits Cazemier, then the nurses interpret this as a torture that patients are forced to go through before they are allowed to die. This brings to mind a sick joke that was being told in hospitals.

Two missionaries are captured by savages. They are taken to the chief who says to the first missionary 'You can choose between *cheechee* or death'. The first missionary says that he would rather have *cheechee* and immediately they grab him, tie him to a pole and proceed to beat him. They then tie him behind a horse and drag him over the ground for a kilometre, during which he loses teeth and other body parts. Finally they throw him down a cliff. The other missionary is terrified as the chief comes to him and says, 'What'll it be for you? *Cheechee* or death?' The missionary answers, 'I didn't think it would ever come to this, but I think I prefer death.' 'Good,' says the chief, 'but a bit of *cheechee* first'.

(Zussman 1992: 111–12)

This is how nurses experience the treatment of some patients. Shortly before Mr Heuvel there was another patient with small-cell lung carcinoma who was admitted for rescue therapy. A thrombocyte deficiency caused by the first course of chemotherapy resulted in a nocturnal pulmonary haemorrhage. She died after a gruesome struggle, leaving the nurses who were involved traumatized.[1]

Explanations

The cases of Mr Heuvel and Frits Cazemier illustrate how doctors and nurses can differ in what they consider to be the best treatment for a particular patient. In what follows I will attempt to explain these differences.

To begin at the beginning, the two groups have different tasks, positions and responsibilities in the social system that is the hospital. Doctors are responsible for the medical-technical aspects of treatment whereas the nurses are responsible for care. They have undergone very different training with their concomitant socialization processes. Different backgrounds and a differential division of labour make for divergent experiences of particular cases. Generally speaking, nurses have a more intensive and more intimate contact with patients. As a result they have different information about the patient. In Chapter 2, I described the smaller social distance between nurses and patients and the way in which nurses are available at difficult moments. Each nurse is responsible for a small number of patients, whereas a doctor may be responsible for a whole ward and have patients on other wards as well.

In the outpatient clinic doctors have relatively short encounters with patients, but over a much more extended period than the nurses on the ward. Moreover, the nurses are involved with the patient during a relatively short

---

1 See The 1997a, Chapter 1 for a description of this patient.

period of 'sea sickness,' as one nurse put it. Patients are admitted to the ward because they are seriously ill. When they improve they are sent home. Nurses do not generally interact with patients in the period in which they are relatively well. Doctors who have patients in their outpatient practice see them in bad times and in good times.

The differences in responsibility are also important. Nurses are not permitted to decide about important issues; doctors *must* decide. Nurses are more dependent on doctors' decisions than vice versa. It was the doctors who decided that Mr Heuvel and Mr Cazemier should be treated. The nurses were not involved in this decision, but they were exposed to its consequences. Indeed, they had to deal with the results of decisions they did not agree with. In this sense nurses are subordinate to doctors.

The other side of the story is that doctors have to bear the burden of responsibility. This makes it easier to understand why they are reluctant to give up treatment. They feel that they cannot deny patients their last chance of cure. By treating him they 'at least tried' to save Frits Cazemier (Tijmstra 1987). Nuland (1995) discusses a number of influential factors that I will mention briefly here.

First, medical culture: doctors have been socialized to think in a medically responsible manner, which emphasizes diagnosis and treatment. Medically responsible interventions are not by definition humane. Second, doctors have the desire to be a *healer*. Third, mutual social control: doctors persevere with treatment because they are worried about criticism by colleagues.

Nurses do not bear responsibility for treatment, but they are confronted by the patient's suffering. Mira Kuipers, who took care of Frits Cazemier when he was more dead than alive and who had to winch him out of bed to weigh him experienced his suffering differently from the doctors who had decided to treat him. She saw the treatment as meaningless torture. Seeing somebody in pain is painful, seeing somebody sad is saddening. It is these resonances of suffering and emotion that make nursing such a burden.[2]

Conflicts between doctors and nurses are often about authority, responsibility, priorities and the division of labour. Nurses often resist through territoriality (Zussman 1992). The way in which Mira Kuipers and her colleagues refused to take Mr Cazemier for his tests is an example of this. All these factors contribute to doctors and nurses having divergent perspectives, from which they then make different judgements about 'doing the right thing'. They also contribute to the criteria that each group uses to determine what 'the right thing' is. The nurse Mira Kuipers had serious doubts about Frits Cazemier's treatment, 'you could just see that he would

---

2 Free translation of a remark by E. Engelhard during a presentation on terminal care at a meeting of the Union for Psychosocial Oncology (NVPO) on 15 March 1996. Many of the doctors I spoke to during this and other studies agreed with this.

not survive the treatment,' she said. This was not convincing evidence for the doctors, though. The important thing for them was to chart the patient's illness, to unravel and objectify it. For them, Frits Cazemier could be cured in theory.

It is a well-known contrast: the doctors looking at the X-rays and laboratory results and declaring that the patient is doing fine, while the nurses appeal for them to come to the bedside to see that the patient is not fine at all. Each group seeks evidence for its own interpretation.

In academic medical training, objective, logical reasoning is central. Doctors have to defend their decisions and legitimacy is based on proof. Doctors may hold an individual opinion, as long as it can be objectified. This is much less important for nurses; they can hold opinions based on individual impressions. Doctors and nurses are each trained in different skills and their professional socialization processes occur separately. This influences their language, their ways of reasoning and the types of language that they are responsive to. Tensions often develop because they do not understand each other's language. Also, because doctors are medically responsible, they have to base their irreversible decisions on more than feeling. In such cases it is easier to retreat to your own disciplinary territory and base your decision on medical criteria.

X-rays and scans

[16 April] Mr Dekker, Mr and Mrs Wiersema, Mr and Mrs Bokjes and Mr Koster and his daughter are waiting for their regular check-ups in the outpatient clinic. Mr Koster and Mr Bokjes have completed their last course of chemotherapy. It is a busy morning. Dr Heller is alone because the other doctors are attending a conference.

Mr Wiersema is the first to be called. When Dr Heller asks how the chemotherapy went, Mr Wiersema immediately answers 'Fine' and makes a thumbs-up sign. As he speaks his eyes dart about nervously. 'I've been a bit more nauseous than last week, but it wasn't too bad,' he says. The picture of him bending over a cardboard kidney dish during most of the past few days comes to my mind. Mr Wiersema enquires about the CT scan that had been made a few days earlier. Dr Heller reads the radiologist's report and mutters 'Good'. Mr and Mrs Wiersema exchange relieved glances. 'Then we're off to the caravan,' he says, putting his arm round his wife's shoulder.

Mr Dekker also enquires about his scan. Dr Heller once again reads the radiologist's report. 'Not very reassuring,' he mumbles, 'a new lesion.' The colour drains from Mr Dekker's face. Dr Heller gets up and hangs the scan on the viewing box next to the previous one. What seems like an interminable silence follows as he examines the scans. 'No,' he concludes finally, turning to Mr Dekker. 'They didn't look properly. That lesion isn't new at all; it's visible on the old scan as well. The radiologist has made a mistake. The scan is okay.' Mr Dekker sighs deeply.

'So can I reassure my wife?' Mr Dekker asks a few times.

'Yes,' Dr Heller answers. 'You certainly can.'

Mr Koster's X-rays are on the viewing box. 'They look good,' says Dr Heller as he compares Mr Koster's lungs before, during and after chemotherapy. 'You can see for yourself,' he says, as he points to a white patch, a small spot and a striped area. He turns to face Mr Koster and his daughter. 'It seems like your lungs are clear. All that's left is some scar tissue.'

'Great,' Mr Koster beams. 'That's good news.'

Dr Heller smiles. 'It certainly is good news,' he says.

'So there's really nothing there?' Mr Koster asks.

'No,' Dr Heller replies. 'There are no lesions visible. Of course, there may still be something there that isn't visible on the X-ray, that you can't see with the naked eye. If just one cell has survived, we wouldn't see it on the X-ray. We'll have to wait and see.

'Before leaving Mr Koster shakes Dr Heller's hand vigorously. 'Thank you for everything, doctor,' he says. Then he asks, 'Aren't you happy with the result?'

'Yes,' Dr Heller answers, nodding. 'It's very good.' Mr Koster looks at his daughter.

'Isn't it wonderful for the doctor,' he asks, 'to have achieved such a success?' She looks at the doctor. 'Dad thinks he's been cured,' she says. 'He thinks he can go back to work.'

'In theory you can do everything,' Dr Heller says, looking at Mr Koster. 'But don't do anything too strenuous. I don't need to see you back here for another six weeks. If there's a problem before then, just call me.'

Partial and complete remission

'That silence with Mr Dekker was awkward,' Dr Heller says later, when we are discussing the day's events. 'That's the problem when it's so busy and you can't prepare properly,' he answers. 'Unfortunately that's all too common; and we can't always rely on the radiologist's report, so we need to check the pictures ourselves as well. Before we see the patient, that is. Patients often spend a long time in the waiting room. There was a good reason for that today, but even when everyone is here, they have to wait for the results of blood tests and deal with administrative hassle.'

'What would you have done if the lesion on Mr Dekker's scan was new?' I ask.

'Then we would have had to stop the current treatment regimen,' he answers. 'If the tumour continues to grow, or lesions appear in other parts of the body, then that means that it has become resistant to treatment. Continuation is then pointless.'

'What are the criteria for deciding that therapy is no longer effective?' I ask.

'There are internationally recognized criteria, developed by the WHO, for deciding whether or not a patient is responding,' Dr Heller explains. 'A measurement on a thorax X-ray gives a rough estimate. A CT-scan is more accurate. There's always a margin of error though, depending on how you do the measurement. You always try to take the largest measurement, to keep error as small as possible. A decrease in tumour size from 1cm to 0.8cm could, in fact, be no decrease at all given the margin of error. It's a question of millimetres. If the tumour shrinks from 10cm to 8cm then there is much less chance that you're mistaken. It was decided that a patient would be defined as a 'complete responder' if the tumour were no longer visible at all. We refer to someone as a 'partial responder' if the tumour has reduced in size by more than 50 per cent. We talk of 'stable disease' if the tumour reduces by less than 50 per cent or increases by less than 50 per cent. It is possible that you see on the X-ray that the tumour has increased in size but that this does not conform to the norms of progression. What is unfortunate is when the tumour clearly decreases in size but just doesn't make the 50 per cent mark. But that's how it is.'

'But if a patient has a complete remission, can the tumour still come back?' I ask.

'Yes,' Dr Heller nods. It's possible that tumour cells are still imperceptibly present. It happens. In the case of X-rays there have to be more than a million cells before you can see them. The same applies to the pathologist. If he says, 'In this sample there are no tumour cells, then that only means that there are less than a thousand cells in a certain area. He can't see less than that.'

'Brigit is cured!'

[19 April] Saturday morning during breakfast the phone rings.

'Anne-Mei, it's Ronald Westra,' a voice says. 'Sorry for disturbing you in the weekend.'

'Hello Ronald,' I answer, surprised. 'How are you both?' I know Ronald and Brigit Westra from the hospital. Brigit is not yet 40 but has recently learned that she has a small-cell lung carcinoma that has metastasized to her brain and bones. She is receiving chemotherapy but having a hard time. Each course sees her bedridden for longer. She has lost a lot of weight. I often sit on her bed chatting. She is worried about the future of her five children. After the third course of chemotherapy the specialist, Dr van Os, had told the couple that he was not sure whether she would be able to cope with another. She had now just completed the fourth course. During their rounds the doctors had been very worried about her condition.

'We've got great news,' I hear Ronald Westra proclaim at the other end of the line. His voice is excited. 'Brigit is cured! I said to her, "We have to tell Anne-Mei"'.

'But,' I stammer. 'What's happened?'

'Well,' Ronald explains, 'on Friday we spoke to Dr van Os. 'He said it was pointless to continue treatment. Yes, those were his exact words: it was pointless. Brigit doesn't need to have any more chemo.'

'Ronald,' I say. 'Why doesn't Brigit need any more chemo?'

'Because she's cured.'

'But didn't they tell you, just a couple of weeks ago, that the chemo had become too much for her, that *that* is why they were planning to stop?' I ask desperately.

'I asked Dr van Os the reason,' Ronald answers. 'And do you know what he answered? He said, 'It is pointless to continue the chemotherapy because we have already achieved the *optimal effect.*' What can 'optimal effect' mean other than cure?'

The generation of optimism about recovery

The optimism about cure that I had observed during previous research inspired the present study. I wondered how this was possible in an era in which the ideology of individual autonomy and self-determination is so dominant. In what follows I will attempt to describe the contributing factors. Chronologically, in the illness trajectory of the patient, the 'relative peace of mind' that I described in Chapter 3 gives way to a certain optimism about recovery. Although patients occasionally mentioned dying shortly after receiving the bad news of their diagnosis, this topic was hardly ever mentioned during therapy. At a certain point the fatal outcome of the illness becomes taboo and patients only tell 'restitution narratives'.[1] The bad news seems to have given way completely to treatment, the solution, 'doing something'.

It is well known that patients find it difficult to remember what the doctor has told them during the bad news interview.[2] It is not only the sick who have to make an effort to remember something they have heard only once. For example, if a doctor wanted to remember more than five per cent of a presentation then he would have to read the text more than once, preferably shortly after the presentation and then again later (Radovsky 1985, cited in Wagener 1987: 1006). And this is an *ordinary* presentation, not one in which it is announced that you are going to die. If it is so difficult for healthy people to absorb information, how difficult must it be for patients and their relatives to absorb information in such an emotionally charged situation as the bad news interview (Wagener 1996: 31)?

Although the doctors I encountered did their best to avoid medical jargon and use everyday language, the language they used was not familiar to the patient and therefore not easy to understand. In addition doctors are, whether intentionally or unintentionally, 'champions of veiled language' (Wagener 1996: 14, my translation). The way in which Dr van Os tells Mr and

---

1 The term 'restitution narrative' is taken from Frank (1995).
2 Ley (1988) has shown that 20–60 per cent of hospital patients do not properly remember the information they have been given.

Mrs Westra that the tumour is progressive is a good example: 'Chemotherapy has already achieved the optimal effect.' But simply saying 'you are not going to get better' sounds much less threatening than 'you are going to die'. This euphemistic use of language is also evident in the jargon that doctors use when talking to each other. In the discussion with Dr Liem, reported in Chapter 2, it is apparent that cure is not an option, so they strive to make patients 'long-term survivors' instead. 'Long' in this case meaning five years. It was easy for me to imagine why patients did not properly understand what the doctors were telling them. The seriousness of the bad news hardly got through to me in the early stages of the study, even though I was not sick myself, not accompanying a sick relative, theoretically aware of the disastrous course of the illness, and familiar with the doctors' academic level of thinking and reasoning.

The 'double message' presented in the bad news interview distracts attention from the bad news itself. Shortly before her husband died, the wife of one patient told me 'The doctor told us how things were. He certainly did. We went into the consulting room and the doctor said that he couldn't cure my husband. He immediately followed this by saying that there *was* something he could do. I thought, 'At least he can do something'. I didn't realize [what the situation really was].' It is not only contradictions in the doctor's spoken words that cause confusion; the same also applies to non-verbal communication. The treatment itself sometimes has a magical aura. Mrs Wiersema described this appositely: 'Dr Liem told us that only seven per cent of the patients are cured. But then he went on to do all kinds of things: chemotherapy, lab tests, radiotherapy, you name it. We thought, "It must be effective, otherwise they wouldn't do it." We gradually developed hope. We thought that he was among the seven per cent. No, we *knew* he was one of them.'[3]

In the case of small-cell lung carcinoma the course of the illness plays a crucial role in the development of hope. As a result of therapy the tumour melts away like snow before the sun. There is a discrepancy between the earlier bad news and what actually happens subsequently. The doctor says, 'It's going well, the therapy is working,' 'there are hardly any lesions visible,' 'your lungs are clear'. The patient can see the tumour shrinking on the X-rays. It is difficult for him to see the developments in proportion. Initially he did not feel sick at all and the white patches on the X-rays were proof of the ominous truth. When this proof 'disappears,' it is difficult not to draw

---

3 For an outsider seven per cent seems like a slim chance. Those who are involved perceive this differently. One of the nurses illustrated this with a personal story. She said that she became angry when she saw how patients pin all hope on that small chance. She said it was almost criminal the way doctors held that 'carrot' before the patient. When she also became a patient in connection with an infertility problem, that one per cent chance suddenly became real for her.

positive conclusions. The effect of therapy *looks just like cure* (The et al. 1996: 2003). In the case of non-small-cell lung carcinoma the tumour seldom disappears completely. The lesions may simply become smaller or remain stable, though still visible. But even these patients had hope. The doctors' explanation that these lesions were not necessarily tumours but might be scar tissue played a role in this.

The way in which the doctor provides information during treatment is an important source of confusion. Doctors describe the leitmotif of the illness, its disastrous outcome, only after diagnosis and before commencing treatment. During the actual treatment they do not return to this topic. They only tell the patient about the treatment, not about what comes after the treatment. The implicit code is that if the patient does not ask about the long-term or the outcome, then the doctor will certainly not mention it. A research fellow who was often critical about the way in which doctors informed their patients, once told me, 'I go along with the patient. I only break down their hope when it is necessary' (i.e. *medically* necessary due to the reappearance of the tumour). That which doctors and patients conspire to ignore, patients tend to forget (de Swaan 1985: 32).

The frame of reference that doctors use when reporting to the patient is the therapy. 'It's going well,' means 'It's going well with the *therapy*'; it means that the therapy is having some effect. Doctors consider this way of informing the patient legitimate, if only because it fits with their interpretation of their role. They are there for the clinical aspects of the illness. 'I'm here for the lungs,' Dr Veerman often said apologetically, and he was not the only specialist who spoke like this. So when doctors tell a patient with a small-cell lung carcinoma that things are going well, they mean they are going well given the situation. For patients these statements often have a completely different meaning. They interpret them as meaning, 'All is well with *me*'. And 'good' is easily interpreted as 'better'. The doctors' use of language supports this kind of interpretation by the patient. The doctor says, 'Your lungs are clear, I don't see any lesions,' and when you look at the X-ray it seems they are right.

I do not want to finish this summing up of factors relating to optimism about cure by pointing an accusatory finger at doctors. Patients interpret what doctors say the way they do because they *want* to get better. Not having any future is distressing. It is not death per se that causes problems for people, but the knowledge that you are going to die (Elias 1990). It is not uncommon that patients listen selectively to doctors and reconstruct reality is a way that is more acceptable to them. The difference in interpretations is dominated by our deeply rooted resistance to mortality and powerlessness in the face of death. As a reflex, various defence mechanisms come into play and patients clutch at every straw (The et al. 1996: 2023). Here hope survives. Everyone who is sick wants to get better; being healthy is the 'normal' state of affairs.

The pessimistic patient as exception

Almost all of the patients with small-cell lung carcinoma (and most of the relatives) I met during my years of research in the Ruysdael Clinic were optimistic about the chances of recovery; both those in my study and those I encountered on the wards or in the consultation rooms. Of course, some were more optimistic than others, or perhaps, some expressed their optimism better than others. However, not all patients were optimistic about recovery.

I met three patients who did not cherish this hope. The first was 48-year-old Mr Boom. I was not really involved in his case. I encountered him occasionally, accompanied by his wife, during outpatient consultations. They talked openly about the pressures on the family and the rapidly approaching time of saying goodbye. The couple were actively discussing what they should do with their joint architecture firm. She was not sure whether she wanted to continue with the business by herself. After one of these consultations Dr Heller was called away and the couple lingered to talk to me. Mrs Boom asked me exactly what I was doing. When I started telling them about communication she interrupted me. 'Very interesting,' she said. 'But have you noticed how patients here think they're going to get better? Lennard spent three weeks on the ward not so long ago and you could just *see* the optimism in the patients there. The doctors say that there's no chance of cure – they told us that as well – but then they go on to say "your lungs are *clear*" and "there are *no more lesions* visible".' Her voice rises in pitch. 'You can see the hope developing.'

The second patient was 68-year-old Mr van der Velde, a recently retired lawyer. From the moment he arrived in the hospital his ideas were clear. He wanted the kind of treatment that would give him some time to finish off important business but not require him to spend a lot of time in hospital. He wanted to be present at the opening of his son's new law firm and wanted to be there when his oldest grandchild started talking. He realized that his life was coming to an end and seemed to accept this. If he could be given these last two experiences then he would be satisfied.

The most obvious similarity between these two patients is their level of education: they were both professional. This is striking, as highly trained patients were under-represented in my study.[4] In fact, these were the only highly educated patients I encountered in my study.

---

4 Mr Post, who was mentioned by Dr Liem in Chapter 2, was a professor in econometrics, and he also did not have a recovery narrative. Mr Post did not live with the hope that he would be cured. Because he did not have a small-cell lung carcinoma it would not be justified to introduce him into the discussion here. Not hoping does not mean refusing therapy. The patients I am describing here were just as motivated to accept treatment as any of the others.

At this point I want to comment on something I mentioned in Chapter 2. More highly educated patients are treated differently by doctors, they receive more and more detailed information about their illness. These patients are more inclined to ask questions, which in turn also generates information. It is therefore possible that the realization of being incurable is not simply a result of having a 'more highly educated ear' but also a result of the doctor's different pattern of providing information. These patients were not only highly educated, they were also professionals of the same standing as the doctor.

There is, however, another category of patients who do not cherish hope. Mrs Rogge, who was 61 years old, was always accompanied by her husband when she came to the outpatient clinic. Sometimes one of her children also came along. When the doctor responded positively to the results of first-line chemotherapy she was obviously pleased. Later, pondering over the X-rays, she said, 'Maybe I will get better then.' The doctor did not reply. Her daughter, a community nurse, intervened. 'Ma,' she said, 'remember what Dr Veerman said during the first consultation?' Mrs Rogge nodded. 'He said that cure was not an option,' the daughter continued, 'and I don't think that has changed in the meantime.' She looked at the doctor for support. He nodded. 'I'm sorry,' he said.

During her illness it was Mrs Rogge's children who reminded her that her illness was incurable. Eventually the patient herself also began to talk of her illness as incurable. Many patients were accompanied by adult children, but none of the others helped their parent to remember the doctor's initial words about the illness being essentially incurable. I think that the background of Mrs Rogge's children played a role: two were nurses and one was a hospital physiotherapist. They were all familiar with the traps inherent in doctor–patient communication.

In this respect they are similar to two of the three patients who refused chemotherapy; they were also familiar with the health care sector. They both realized immediately that the treatment was palliative and that there was no hope of cure. The third patient who refused chemotherapy had knowledge of the disease and knew the inevitable outcome.

The case of Mrs Rogge illustrates that hope of cure is not an individual but a *collective* affair. Mrs Rogge wanted to hope, and if she could find a straw to clutch in the words of the doctor she did. She did not have a chance to develop that hope further, however, because her children did not allow her to. Not only were they professionally familiar with the disease and the tendency of patients to hope for a cure, but they were also present during all the important meetings and consultations. When laboratory results were discussed Mr and Mrs Rogge were always accompanied by one of their children and as a result they knew exactly what the doctor had said.

The similarity between Mrs Rogge's children and the nurses in the Ruysdael Clinic was their knowledge of the illness, the difference was that the Clinic nurses were not present during consultations with the doctor and thus had no means of intervening directly. When patients are hopeful about cure and say that they derive this hope from what the doctor has told them then the nurses can only speculate as to what the doctor actually said. As a result they will be reluctant to say anything about the course of the illness. They are not likely to correct what the patient has said and as a result the patient has scope to develop hope further. The tragedy is that by not contradicting the patient, the nurses contribute to the development of hope. If nurses did participate in meetings between doctor and patient, like Mrs Rogge's children, they would be in a position to discuss with the patient what the doctor had said in a meaningful way.

I carried out another study in the peripheral Randstad Hospital. I was investigating decisions at the end of life on the Intensive Care ward, but also regularly spoke to doctors and nurses from the lung and oncology departments. I noticed that the oncology nurses were present during most of the oncologist's consultations with patients, including bad news interviews. It was striking that both doctor and nurses talked about *joint consultations*. The nurse generally had another meeting shortly after that with the doctor in which they went over what had been said. The nurse often had the patient repeat what the doctor had said. They also saw how patients' optimism about cure developed, but they were able to correct the patients' misinterpretations of what the doctor had said.

Optimism about recovery develops during patients' interaction with their social environment and is therefore a collective affair. If the patients' interlocutors are unwilling to participate in this process, as in the case of Mrs Rogge and the Randstad Hospital nurses, then there is much less chance of optimism developing.

'What doctors really tell patients'

[20 April] Monday morning, between outpatient consultations, I stroll into the coffee room where Mark van Rossum is working on the shift timetable.

'How are things?' he asks, without looking up. I'm still unhappy about the phone conversation with Ronald Westra.

'Okay,' I say. 'Yesterday something happened that I'm still thinking about.' I tell him the story.

Mark puts his papers aside and listens attentively. 'That's something we nurses experience all the time,' he says when I have finished. 'The first time I experienced something like that was before I worked here. My brother's father-in-law had a small-cell lung carcinoma. He was being treated by Guido Liem and Marcel Heller. I clearly remember that the family were to go out to dinner. I asked what they were celebrating. Well, the father-in-law had just completed his first course of chemotherapy and he was cured. That's what the celebration was for. I didn't doubt for a moment, but when I came to work here I saw him with a recurrence. It was a huge disappointment; the family hadn't anticipated this. I remember thinking that there was something wrong somewhere; either they had been given the wrong information or they had interpreted things wrongly.

'I've noticed that patients sometimes think they are cured. These days I keep an eye open for that kind of thing. It's really terrible, organizing parties. Okay if they're going out to dinner because the first course of treatment has been completed. But not to celebrate cure. You know, the worst thing about that group of patients is that you can predict exactly how things are going to end. Then the next couple reports to the outpatient clinic . . . Sometimes I really worry about it. It makes me miserable, every time you hear them say "We have to tackle this thing together, we have to fight on".'

'Do you have the impression that most of the patients in this category have hope?'

'Yes, definitely. Now that I've been here longer I'm less afraid to ask patients what the doctor has said. It's a real struggle finding out whether the patient knows that he is fatally ill and that the treatment is only palliative.'

Communication between doctors and nurses

'Then I got in touch with the doctors themselves,' Mark continues. 'But I still didn't find out exactly what they were telling patients. There was a reason for this. There was a woman with small-cell lung carcinoma who came to us for her chemotherapy. I don't know what they had been told, but she and her family were convinced that she was going to get better. Five courses of treatment and that's it, they said. That's not it at all, I thought. I tried to influence the conversation but that didn't work. I told Dorien Meulman that I had the impression that nothing of what Dr Veerman had said seemed to have come across. Dorien talked to them a few times and repeated what the doctor had said. It was a tremendous shock for them. After that incident we had a meeting. We demanded that the doctors tell us exactly what they tell patients. But even then it's difficult to know exactly what they say and how they say it. They say things like "If I don't treat you then you'll be dead in a few months, but I can do something for you". Then the whole chemotherapy process follows.

'What doctors don't realize sufficiently is that patients want to get better. I think that patients don't get enough time to get used to the idea that there is no treatment that is going to keep them alive, that they are going to die. Doctors claim that they have informed patients, but I doubt it because of what I hear from the patients themselves. They make plans to go on holiday when "everything is over". Then when they get a recurrence it takes them completely by surprise. I ask the doctors to explain to me why it is that patients are so disappointed if everything has been explained to them, but they just say, "It's a normal human reaction." People always respond to hope, but it's not only the patient who's responsible for such disappointment, it's also the fault of the counselling. I doubt whether they give the patient sufficient room to respond. If you say to the patient, "I can't cure you. If we don't do anything then you'll be dead in three months, but we can treat you," that doesn't give the patient much room to respond. And they easily forget the first part of what the doctor said.'

'So how could things be improved?' I ask.

'I think it would be good if there was somebody present during those discussions, a nurse for example, who can respond to what was said. The best thing would be if the doctors invited us to those discussions routinely. That would enable us to deal with the patients much more adequately because you know exactly what was said. What happens now is that they have their first interview and then they end up coming to us for their treatment, and in between there has been no counselling at all.'

'What do you think of the communication in the outpatient clinic?' I ask.

'The lines of communication are so short, but sometimes it's a real mess. Patients often have to wait a long time. Sometimes they come for the results of a scan but the results haven't arrived yet. Then I think to myself, "Damn it, get up out of your chair and go and find them, or don't make the appointment so early, or plan it a few days later". You know how it is when you're waiting for results of tests in hospital, people get all worked up. Doctors tend to forget that, they seem to turn off their capacity for empathy.'

'You say that nurses have intensive contact with patients,' I say. 'Doctors have a different kind of intensive contact with patients. Doctors and nurses work closely together year in and year out, but you still don't communicate with each other about such fundamental things as how the bad news is given, even though you get frustrated about it.'

'We've tried to organize a forum for discussion with the lung oncologists,' says Mark, 'but it came to nothing. I'm not sure what went wrong.'

'Can you see why I'm surprised?' I ask.

'It *is* surprising,' the nurse chuckles. '*Very* surprising. I agree. It's a pity because we could help each other. In situations like that we could be very complementary. You'd think doctors would be interested to know what went on outside the consultation room. Patients sometimes give the impression that they've understood everything, but then when they come to us we realize they haven't understood a thing. In cases like that we should be able to discuss and guide the patient together. Yes, it's a pity that doesn't happen.'

'Why do you attach so much importance to patients understanding exactly what is happening?' I ask.

'I think it's important so that patients can use the time still remaining as fully as possible. It is terrible if you die and didn't get to say things to your partner that you wanted to say, or do things you wanted to do. Fortunately there are people who do that. Rene and Linda Hartog, for example. They met each other four years ago. Rene was sick for the last two years. Linda said that she has never had such intensive contact with anyone as she did with Rene during those two years. She said that you don't even have that kind of contact after 25 years of marriage. They were well aware of the situation and they knew that he was going to die. They had hope, of course, but when the recurrence came they were ready. When the end came it was hard, but they were prepared. To make proper use of the time that remains you need to be counselled properly and convinced that there isn't much time left.'

Involuntary play acting

I am standing in the ward kitchen with one of the nurses, Carola Vroon.
   'You've had a lot to do with Mr Wiersema haven't you?' she asks.
   'Yes, why?'
   'Well, a while ago, when he was here on the ward for his chemotherapy, I had a chat with him. He said that things were fine, the X-rays looked good and there were no more lesions visible. I was surprised and didn't know what to say.'
   'Does that sort of thing happen more often?' I ask.
   'Yes, it's not the first time. It's something that gets me thinking. Those are really difficult moments. Patients are admitted for a blood transfusion or for chemo-therapy and claim they are cured. It's happened a couple of times. It makes me feel as though I'm being dishonest toward the patient.'
   'As though you're lying by not saying anything?' I suggest.
   'Yes,' she nods. 'It's like involuntary play acting, and it worries me. When I had worked here for a while I realized that most of the patients who receive chemotherapy don't get better. But it's not discussed openly. And I noticed that patients cherish the hope of cure. At first I wondered whether I was interpreting things properly. I did some reading and then did the oncology course and I realized that the treatment wasn't curative at all but only palliative.'
   'But patients do hope they will be cured,' I say.
   'Yes,' Carola nods. 'When I discuss the treatment with them they often say they have no choice. When I ask them what they mean they answer that if they don't accept treatment then they will die. I don't dare to tell them that they're going to die anyway.'
   'Maybe it sounds a bit tasteless,' I say, 'but why is it so important for patients to know exactly what the situation is? Maybe it's easier for them to cope if they have hope.'
   'Hope is important, I agree,' she says. 'Maybe it's a cliché, but hope really does keep you going, and you shouldn't deprive patients of their hope. It's a difficult issue.'
   'But you think honesty is more important?'
   'Yes.'
   'Why?'
   'If someone . . . If patients really know what the situation is then they are in a better position to say goodbye, to achieve closure. If you are too focused on completing the chemotherapy, not being defeatist, not shedding a tear then

you're blocked and only focused on the future. If, on the other hand, you admit to yourself that there's nothing more that can be done, then you can concentrate on what you want to say to others in the time that remains, what still remains to be enjoyed. Then you are more consciously focused on the present.

[3 May] 'He's having a hard time,' Mrs Wiersema tells me when she comes to pick up her husband. Just like the previous occasion, Mr Wiersema can hardly wait to go home. He has not even bothered to shower; he will do that at home, in his own bathroom. Mrs Wiersema has made a large pan of soup so that he can build up his strength. It is the only food he still feels like eating.

Consequences: the nurses' frustration

Mark van Rossum and Carola Vroon are concerned that doctors deprive patients of the opportunity to achieve closure through inadequate counselling. They feel that awareness of death is the first step toward good death (see also Kellehear 1992). Nurses complain that it is difficult to care for patients who are not aware of their situation. Patients do not always explicitly say that they think they are going to get better, but their euphoric mood and plans for the future suggest that they do. The obvious question here is why nurses do not inform patients themselves. Moreover, if the doctors claim that they tell patients the truth then it should be relatively easy for nurses to simply confirm this. But that is not how things work in practice.

It is formally the job of the doctor and not the nurse to inform patients about their illness. Nurses do not correct what doctors have said about diagnosis or prognosis. The only authoritative information that is given during treatment comes from the specialist or, more precisely, the specialist-in-charge. Nurses are expected to remain silent about what has not been mentioned and the fact that it has not been mentioned. It is for this reason that nurses continually attempt to find out what the patient has been told, so that they know what they are allowed to discuss with the patient. And also what has been withheld so they know what they should not mention (de Swaan 1985: 32).

Things are still more complicated, however. Even when doctors are open about a patient's prospects, the way in which they inform the patient can carry subtle meanings that are not easy to convey to others. It is not so much a question of whether the doctors tell the truth but of how much of it they tell and how they present it (The et al. 1996: 2021). The exact terminology used and the indirect verbal and non-verbal suggestions are important, but cannot be easily summarized later in a few words (de Swaan 1985: 49). While at the same time the frequent, low-threshold communication between patients and nurses inclines patients to talk to nurses and ask them questions about their illness.

I want to make a few remarks at this point. Firstly about the causal connection which the nurses assume exists between the doctors' counselling and the patients' interpretation of their situation. I think it is rather simplistic to assume that patients' interpretations are determined solely by what doctors tell them. Of course doctors should be clear and repeat what they have said to make sure patients understand, but patients are also participants in this interaction. Patients might sometimes not understand what doctors have told them because they do not want to understand. Being told that you have an incurable illness is so traumatic that it triggers defence mechanisms. No matter how good the doctor's counselling is, if patients are not yet ready to receive that information then they will not interpret it properly.

Narratives about recovery and the future can be a goal in themselves. Making plans for holidays is a pleasant activity, even if you know that the holiday will never materialize. Why should patients be deprived of the pleasure of such dreams?

It is also important to distinguish between the optimism that patients express and the optimism that they really have. It is possible that patients are aware, deep down inside, of the disastrous outcome of their illness but do not want to talk or even think about it. This will depend on the extent to which they want to share their awareness of the illness and its prognosis with others.

In other words patients can express hope of cure differently to different people. I sometimes heard patients talking to nurses about getting cured and then saw them, a few minutes later, nodding as the doctor told them that it was only a question of time before the tumour reappeared. It is quite possible that patients reveal different levels of consciousness about their illness depending on their interlocutor. It is easier for patients to express narratives of hope to the nurses, who were not present during the bad news interview and are not in a position to contradict what the patient says, than to present these to the doctor.

There are also other reasons for patients expressing hope to some and not to others. Patients can present an optimistic picture because they do not want to embarrass the person they are talking to, or they do not want the person to feel sorry for them, or they do not want to endanger relationships with people who are important to them. These motives can all lead to positive impression management (Kellehear 1992: 77).

6 Reflection and anxiety

'So I can tell my wife you're satisfied?'

[21 April] Both Mr Wiersema and Mr Dekker are attending the outpatient clinic for blood tests. Depending on the results, they will be offered a fourth course of chemotherapy. As I look round the waiting room Dr Heller calls Mr Wiersema into his office. I walk across and sit next to Mr Dekker.

'Yesterday I went to see the pastor,' he said. 'We discussed life and death.'

'Is the issue exercising you?' I ask carefully.

'Of course,' he answers. 'I'm scared and I think about such things. I've been asking myself why this has happened to me. But because of the accident and the death of Rietje's sister, I no longer feel invulnerable. I no longer think that these things only happen to others. But I do want to get better,' he says, with determination in his voice. 'That's why I'm persevering with this treatment.'

We sit for a while in silence. 'If things don't go right,' he continues after a while, 'then there will be plenty of time left to worry. If I have, say, another two years to go and I start worrying now, then we won't have a very nice time during those two years, will we? Listen, when you are given the diagnosis your whole world collapses. But I don't want to burden others with my problems. I want to make things as pleasant as possible for my family, especially for my wife. She's suffered enough already. My illness hasn't been good for her.' We chat on for a while. Then suddenly he pulls my sleeve. 'Which doctor do you like the best?' he asks.

'They all have their good and bad points,' I suggest.

He laughs. 'You don't want to tell me?'

I laugh without committing myself.

'I like Dr Heller,' he says. 'He's nice. When I'm on the ward he always comes along in the late afternoon and chats. He's not remote from the patients. And his hair is always unkempt.' I look up and see the object of our discussion coming toward us, with Mr and Mrs Wiersema on his heels.

'Klaas, my blood isn't as it should be,' Mr Wiersema informs his fellow patient. 'No chemo for me today. I have to come back next week and have it checked again.'

'Too bad, Joop.' Mr Dekker gives him a pat on the shoulder.

'Are you coming?' Dr Heller asks Mr Dekker. Once inside the office Dr Heller asks, without looking up from the papers in front of him, 'Tell me, why are you two always laughing?'

Mr Dekker replies disarmingly, 'Doctor, we were just talking about you.'

'Really,' Dr Heller replies, looking at us across the table. 'I hope it wasn't anything bad.'

'Doctor,' Mr Dekker says, 'I'd like to bring you a present, a cake or something.'

'That's really not necessary,' replies Dr Heller. 'I do my job and I get paid for it.'

'I know,' replies the patient, 'but I would like to bring you something.'

After chatting for a while longer the doctor examines Mr Dekker and finds that he cannot undergo chemotherapy either. He tells Mr Dekker that they will do another blood test next week. Then Mr Dekker asks, 'Doctor, how am I really doing?'

'Well,' answers Dr Heller, 'we're halfway through the treatment and up to now everything is fine. The therapy is having an effect, but I don't want to commit myself.' He looks in Mr Dekker's file. 'You had metastases in the lymph nodes, and that makes treatment a lot more difficult. We shall have to see how things develop.'

'But doctor,' says Mr Dekker, posing his usual closing question, 'can I tell my wife you are satisfied?'

'Yes,' Dr Heller nods. 'You can tell her that.'

Mr Wiersema perseveres

[28 April] The blood of the two patients is now found to have recovered sufficiently for a new course of chemotherapy. They share a room on the ward, the sun in shining, the mood is merry. During visiting hours the two men and their wives are sitting out on the balcony enjoying the sun, together with Mr Fresco, Mr Bokjes and Mr Wessels, three other patients with the same illness. When I arrive, Mr Dekker asks in a loud voice whether I could nip round to the supermarket for a crate of beer.

[29 April] In the morning Mr Wiersema is nauseous and this will last until the end of his stay on the ward. He does not feel like company and looks pale. When I pass by he asks me to come and sit on his bed.

'You're having a hard time,' I suggest. He nods. 'Everything will be okay, everything will be okay,' he keeps mumbling. 'I'm sure the tumour has gone. The first three courses of chemo got rid of most of it. Now it's just that last bit. This course should be enough for that. Natasha says I shouldn't even be coming to the hospital anymore, but I come anyway. Everything's going to be okay with me, and it's going to be okay with Dekker as well. I'm sure of that.'

'You get on well with Mr Dekker, don't you?'

He nods. 'Klaas is a good comrade.' We phone each other now and then to see how the other is doing. Haneke and Rietje like it that way. It enables us to discuss things, you see?'

'You know,' he continues in a conspiratorial tone. 'My sister has been going to this faith healer for years, for all kinds of ailments. Not so long ago he asked her, "Is there someone in your family who is seriously ill?" My sister was surprised and said, "Yes, my brother". He asked her to bring him a photo of me. He held his hand over the photo and said, "your brother is nauseous, but that's not the problem; the problem is in his chest. He will get better if he drinks radiated water every day". He didn't even know me,' Mr Wiersema says. 'Amazing, isn't it?'

'Radiated water?'

'Yes, he has these bottles of water that he radiates himself with his hands. That's what gives it its healing power. I drink a glass every evening before going to bed. I'm supposed to drink a glass every morning as well, but I'm not keen on water first thing in the morning, so I give that one a miss.'

'Very interesting, but tell me, aren't you worried at all?' I ask. I am thinking about Mr Dekker's visit to the pastor.

'Not at all,' he answers resolutely. 'I don't worry at all. What use is it? When I was told that I was sick it was difficult, but now I'm persevering.' His eyes dart around the room. 'I have to get back to work, don't I?'

Mrs Dekker is worried

[24 May] The day before Mr Dekker was due in hospital for his fifth course of chemotherapy he reports to the emergency room saying that he had coughed up blood while he was out shopping. X-rays are made but the doctor cannot see anything unusual and discharges him. During the night he coughs up blood again. His wife and Vera are very worried. Mr Dekker phones the doctor on duty, who says that Mr Dekker must decide himself whether it is serious enough to come to the hospital. He comes, mainly to satisfy his family.

[25 May, early morning] Before rounds the doctors are discussing the patients. 'And then we have Mr Dekker,' Dr Rutgers says. 'Born in '43, has a small-cell lung carcinoma, extended disease, in the right upper lobe with metastases in the lymph nodes. He was due to start his fifth course of chemo today. Yesterday he had a *haemoptysis*. Called me a number of times yesterday and last night. We've done a bronchoscopy.' He hangs a series of X-rays on the viewing box. 'A tremendous response to chemotherapy,' he reads from the report. 'After a single course the node in the neck had disappeared completely. The tumour has reduced by 80 per cent. Great result.'

[25 May, afternoon] Mr Dekker comes to the reception desk where I am sitting reading. He looks dejected.

'Anne-Mei, have you got a minute, please?' he asks. I follow him to a quiet corner. 'My blood's not good again,' he says. 'They're sending me home without chemo. Dr Rutgers says maybe next week. Do you think I should speak to Dr Heller? Rietje is upset, and we know him much better. She's outside with Johan, crying. I'd like Dr Heller to explain everything to her. Can you ask him?'

I promise to do my best. In the doctors' office I find Dr Kooiman, a junior doctor, who had first informed Mr Dekker that he had cancer. Dr Kooiman is willing to explain things to Mrs Dekker. We go to my office. Mr and Mrs Dekker, Dr Kooiman and I sit on the old office chairs, Johan sits on the television. Mrs Dekker looks sad, but she has stopped crying. Mr Dekker occasionally shoots a nervous glance at her.

Dr Kooiman says there is no cause for worry. The bronchoscopy went well and the malignant cells have reduced.

'I'm so scared that delaying treatment will allow the cancer to grow,' says Mrs Dekker. 'And that when you do finally do it, it won't work.'

The doctor shakes his head. 'You shouldn't worry about that. Listen, when someone has a broken leg that has been set, he also feels some pain and irritation. It's a sign that the leg is healing. That's how you should see things,' Dr Kooiman explains.

'Yes, but Joop Wiersema isn't coughing up blood,' Mrs Dekker responds.

'I trust this hospital fully,' Mr Dekker interrupts. His voice in hard. 'I put myself in your hands. I'll cooperate with whatever you want to do. I see it this way: you know what is best for me. I don't have any complaints about the treatment.' Dr Kooiman nods. 'I don't want to worry,' Mr Dekker continues. 'If I don't believe I'm going to get better then I won't.'

The doctor spends some time trying to reassure Mr and Mrs Dekker. After he has left, Mrs Dekker says to me, 'Klaas doesn't talk about his illness. Because of my poor health he always goes to the hospital alone. He never tells me exactly what the doctor has said. I have to squeeze the information out of him. When he comes home and I ask him how things went he always answers, "Good, the doctor is satisfied, and that is the important thing." And I have to make do with that.'

'Klaas wants to go on holiday, *now*'

[3 June] I am sitting on the ward balcony, drinking tea with Mr and Mrs Dekker. They have just given me a present, a large box of chocolates. There is also a card, on which they have written, 'Thank you for everything.'

'I've had a card from Brigit,' says Mr Dekker suddenly. Brigit Westra had been in the bed next to Mr Dekker's when he was first admitted. She had been in a 'dip' after her last course of chemotherapy. The Dekkers had visited her often when she was in hospital. 'They can't do anything more for her,' Mr Dekker says. 'It's the end.'

'I know,' I answer. 'It's terrible.'

I recall Dr Veerman telling Brigit and her husband, after the second-line chemotherapy, that the tumour in her lung was growing again and that it had spread throughout her body.

'The tumour has become resistant to the chemotherapy,' Dr Veerman had said. Brigit bowed her head. She had felt for some time that the end was near. She often talked about having dreams of her own funeral, with Ronald and the children walking behind her coffin. 'And every time the sun is shining, but the girls are wearing different dresses,' she told me. The news was a terrible shock for her husband. I saw the panic in his eyes.

'Are you just going to let us go like this?' he asked, when Dr Veerman had finished. His voice sounded aggressive.

Brigit sighed deeply. 'Ronald,' she tried to calm him down.

'You can't just let us go like this,' he repeated.

'I'm sorry that I've had to tell you this,' Dr Veerman tried to apologize. 'But I have to tell you what your position is.'

'But what are we supposed to do? You can't just leave it at that. What are we to do? Just go home?' The panic gradually gave way to incredulity and despair.

'I'm sorry but I can't really do very much for you now?' Dr Veerman said. Mr Westra did not reply.

'Do you have children?' Dr Veerman asked.

'Five. The youngest is nine, the oldest turned 16 last week,' Brigit replied quietly.

Dr Veerman sighed audibly. 'We have a social worker that you could talk to,' he said. 'Problem is, she only works in the hospital. She can't do home visits. It might be better if you talk to your GP. He can put you in contact with the home care people. I think that it would be better for me to hand you over to him. I can't do any more for you than he can. I'll phone him and up-date him on what we've discussed. I'm sorry, but I can't do much more for you.'

'I'm here mainly for the lungs,' he added, after a pause.

When they got to the reception desk Ronald Westra burst into tears. Mark van Rossum took them to one of the small offices at the end of the corridor.

Later that day I had coffee with Mark. He was fond of Brigit and thought the developments were terrible.

'Brigit is great,' he told me. 'She's one of those patients who shouldn't be allowed to die. She has a hard time with Ronald. He just doesn't want to face reality. She's resigned. She told me recently that she didn't really want to hold on until the bitter end. She's only had the last chemo for Ronald and the children.

That sort of thing happens sometimes. Patients feel that the end is near, they seem to exude calm, but their relatives aren't ready yet, just like Ronald. It's understandable though. Brigit only has to die, Ronald and the children remain behind afterwards. They have to continue with their lives, and that's more difficult.'

'Klaas wants to go on holiday,' Mrs Dekker's voice brings me back to the ward balcony. 'He's suddenly decided he wants to go on holiday.'
'What a good idea,' I reply. 'You should go.'
'We've never been away together,' Mr Dekker explains. 'It's something we must do sooner or later.'
'I'd like to go on holiday,' his wife adds. 'But not *this* summer. Next year we'll have been married 30 years. That would be a good time to go on holiday.'
'But I want to go *this* summer,' Mr Dekker insists. 'I want to enjoy things *now*.'
His wife smiles. 'Next year you'll have recovered from the chemo. Isn't it a much better idea to go then?'

'Are terminally ill patients allowed to stay in the hospital until they die?' I ask nurse Chrisje Gotschalk as we clean up in the ward kitchen.
She sighs.
'It happens,' I answer myself. 'Patients do die in hospital.'
'We're geared to postponing death,' she says. 'Keeping people on this side of death as long as possible. Chemo and hope, that's what it's all about. Yesterday Mr Frigge, a man with a small-cell lung carcinoma, came for a blood transfusion,' she continues. 'He was in good shape; still alive two years after the diagnosis. He's enjoying that extra bit of time. But there are also those who get really sick from the chemo. And then I wonder whether it's all worth it. We nurses often talk of postponing the execution. It's better to say goodbye now, rather than later when you're too sick. Not to mention the waste of money.'
'It's easy to judge when you're a healthy spectator,' I say. 'What would you do if you were in that situation? Perhaps you would also grab the chance.'
'Exactly, you grab every straw,' she answers. 'You keep hoping. When I see Dekker and Wiersema, I often think that they are aware of what's really happening. The hope makes them feel better. But they're still vulnerable.'

Mr Koster reflects on his life

[12 June] I visit Mr Koster at home so that I can interview him. Mrs Koster died ten years ago and Mr Koster lives on a farm with his three daughters and a son-in-law. When I arrive he is waiting for me in front of the house, leaning on his walking stick. Walking has become difficult for him, even with a stick. We greet each other and he shows me around the farm. We go inside and the house smells clean; the eldest daughter is doing spring-cleaning. We sit in the living room adjacent to the kitchen. When I take my tape recorder from my bag Mr Koster suggests we move to another room. I raise my eyebrows questioningly.

'The reception room,' he explains. 'That's where I see the doctor and the vicar.' We move to the reception room, where Sandra brings us coffee and cake.

Mr Koster is finding things difficult. When he speaks of his late wife he has to continually wipe tears from his eyes with his sleeve. His hands tremble so badly that he has to hold his coffee cup with both hands. His nerves have been affected by the chemotherapy. As we speak his wig gradually slips further forward. He tries his best to make everything seem normal. It makes me sad. He says that he had not thought much about his illness during his last stay in the hospital. He was past all that; the messages coming from the doctors are without exception positive. The side effects of the chemo are unpleasant, but the cancer is no longer causing him any problems. He repeats once again his story of Dr Heller raising his arms in the air and exclaiming, 'Mr Koster, there's been a miracle, your lungs are clear, you are cured!'

Of late Mr Koster has been occupied with things other than his illness. His illness has formed the pretext for thinking about his life, about the death of his wife, the relationship with his children, and his work. Because of his illness he has come to see things differently. He had always worked hard, though sometimes he wondered why he bothered. Anyway, at least the children had grown up properly. But he is lonely. He never meets women in the village. Perhaps he should place a contact advert in the paper. He has realized that he should start thinking about himself as well. He is going to do things differently in future. He is also going to organize his financial affairs differently.

At the end of the afternoon we move back to the living room and drink a soda. Sandra joins us. When he leaves the room for a moment she tells me that he is not doing so well.

'He's not getting better; he's so weak. I spend a lot of time taking care of him. He keeps saying that he's fine, but I doubt it. He hardly ever goes outside.'

'What do you think will happen next?' I ask.

'Well,' she replies. 'At first, when dad first heard that he had cancer, we all thought that he would die soon. That's what the doctor had said. But then during the therapy we kept getting positive messages from the hospital. A few months ago dad was in hospital and Dr Heller was so impressed with the X-rays that he threw his arms in the air. He said that dad's lungs were completely clear. So we began to hope.'

Caught between optimism and fear

Small-cell lung carcinoma follows a dynamic course. This applies not only to the illness itself, with the explosive growth of the tumour and the tremendous response to treatment, but also to the related emotional response of the patient. In Part 2, I describe how, after having received their death sentence, patients gradually recover, mentally, during chemotherapy. During this period of 'relative mental calm' there develops, partly as a result of the positive messages coming from the doctors, an atmosphere of optimism among patients and their relatives. This leads to the hope of cure, which gradually comes to be expressed more and more explicitly. In this phase of their illness patients often report having been told by the doctor that they are 'cured'. The mass character of this optimism among patients with small-cell lung carcinoma is striking; it is only the odd patient who does not cherish and express this hope. Hope is accompanied by joy and this gives them the strength to face treatment.

However, as I have shown in Chapter 6, there is not only optimism. During therapy patients deteriorate physically and they feel themselves gradually getting weaker. Even after they have had chemotherapy they do not recover completely; they never regain the level of wellbeing that they had before. There is a discrepancy between the positive messages emanating from the doctors and the visibly good results of therapy on the one hand, and they way they actually feel on the other. During the bad news interview patients often do not feel sick, but based on the X-rays the doctor tells them that they are sick. After chemotherapy the opposite occurs: the doctor says that things look fine on the X-rays but the patient often does not feel well at all. This is all very confusing and alienating for patients: they cannot trust their own bodies.

Patients are optimistic, or rather, they *claim* to be optimistic, while at the same time they are obviously concerned. Or, to put it differently, the mood that one would expect in a patient who really expects to get better or who has really been cured, is absent. So Mr Koster says that he is cured, but he does not behave at all like someone who has just experienced a miracle. He doesn't feel well and he is dejected. Although Mr Wiersema claims not to be concerned, he is now drinking radiated water in addition to his visits to Natasha. Both patients insist that they are fine, but they do not sound convincing. The contrast between the hope that patients claim to cherish and their rapidly deteriorating physical condition and emotional mood gradually increases. In this phase of the illness the mood of hope is no longer unequivocal. Patients and their partners are worried.

There is also another emotional state that is problematic. At the start of each course of chemotherapy Mr Dekker and Mr Wiersema caused a riot on the ward; loud laughter emanated from their room. Each subsequent sojourn on the ward was louder and jollier than the last, until they became almost euphoric. It is as though they could only compensate for their fear by making a lot of noise. The nurses notice that patients in this phase of their illness are often unnaturally jolly and that this contrasts radically with the mood shortly after diagnosis.

In this period differences between the individual patients also become more pronounced. Mr Dekker is obviously worried when he hears that Brigit Westra is dying. He suddenly decides he wants to go on holiday. It is as though he has started to realize what the near future holds for him. He expresses his concerns much more clearly to me than does Mr Wiersema. He tells me that he has discussed life and death with the pastor, and that since his wife's accident he sees life differently; he has realized that he is vulnerable. A similar confession from Mr Wiersema would be unthinkable. It is possible, of course, that Mr Wiersema is going through the same process as Mr Dekker, but that he does not or cannot share this with those close to him. On the surface at any rate the fatal outcome of his illness appears not to exercise him. When they are in the hospital both Mr and Mrs Wiersema have a positive attitude regarding his prospects; she seems to share his optimism.

Not all couples share the same emotions, however. Mrs Dekker, for example, does not share her husband's nascent realization of his impending end. He tries, subtly, to protect her. Because she does not accompany him to the hospital, she is dependent on him for information, and Mr Dekker is economical with the provision of information, simply telling her that things are fine and that the doctor is satisfied. At the end of every consultation Mr Dekker asks the doctor whether he can tell his wife that things are okay, and when the doctor agrees then this absolves him from telling his wife, in his own words, exactly what has transpired during the consultation. When they say that things are fine, the doctors are not lying. They are, after all, only responsible for the clinical aspects of the illness, as Dr Veerman pointed out to the Westras. Doctors recognize that illness is accompanied by psychosocial problems, but they do not see it as their task to find solutions. For them the clinical aspect – treatment – is central (de Swaan 1985: 30) and that is how their words have to be interpreted. When they tell patients that things are fine, they mean that at that moment *treatment* is having the desired result. However, from the perspective of the patient and his family, 'fine' means that *everything* is fine, that they are going to get better.

Brigit and Ronald Westra were another couple who did not share the same realization of approaching death. In their case, as in most other cases I observed, it was the patient who felt death approaching while the partner denied and repressed. Contrary to Mrs Dekker, Ronald Westra was not kept in the dark by his partner. He was present during all consultations but did not want to know what the situation really was. It was only when the doctor said, quite literally, that she was dying, that he seemed to realize what was happening. Mrs Dekker became anxious in a much earlier stage of her husband's illness, due to the contradictory messages she was receiving: on the one hand the positive messages from the doctor as relayed by her husband and on the other his visibly deteriorating condition.

The optimism described in Chapter 5 is real, but at the time there is much evidence that patients and their partners are also worried about the future. They live with hope and fear simultaneously.

PART III

Variations on a recurrence

7 Recurrence

Mr Dekker

[18 August] After my leave I am working in my office in the Ruysdael Clinic when there is a loud knock at the door. The small office is full when I have let in Mr Dekker and Johan. The greetings are warm. I wasn't present during rounds that morning and they had heard from Dr Heller that I was back. Mr Dekker has been out with his stepson and they tell me about their adventures.

'How are things otherwise?' I ask when they have finished.

'Fine,' Mr Dekker says. 'Everything is fine. The cancer's gone; there's nothing left on the X-rays. But I feel worse after the therapy than I did before. I've got numb fingers. Everything is weaker.' He shrugs. He is as friendly and as noisy as ever, and I am pleased to see him.

'And how's your wife?' I ask.

'Fine,' he nods.

'Say hello to her,' I say.

'I will,' he says. 'Why don't you call in to see us one day? Rietje would love that.' He pats me on the shoulder. 'And so would we, wouldn't we Johan?' The lad nods.

'I'd love to,' I say.

'So when are you coming?' he asks. We arrange for a couple of weeks later.

'Will you stay for dinner?' he asks.

'That I can't refuse.'

[27 August] Four days before our arranged meeting I phone the Dekkers to confirm. Johan calls Mr Dekker to the phone and when he speaks his voice sounds strange. At first I think it's the telephone. When I ask him how he's feeling he at first puts on a brave face and says that he is fine, but soon admits that he is not well at all.

'What's wrong?' I ask.

'My voice is so strange,' he says. 'As though I've had too much to drink. People stare at me when I talk, and that's unpleasant. I can't write anymore either. And I can't cycle.' His voice gets more excited. 'I'm unsteady when I stand.'

'When's your next appointment?' I ask.

'In three weeks. Ach, it's probably a side effect of the therapy.'

'It's nothing really,' I hear Mrs Dekker's voice in the background.

'Rietje wants to speak to you,' Mr Dekker says and passes the telephone to his wife.

'It's nothing,' she says, almost crying. 'But his voice is funny and he can't write. And if you could see how funny he walks. It's making him so unsure of himself.

'How long has this been going on?' I ask.

'More than a week.'

'I think you have to go to the hospital earlier,' I say. 'You have to phone and bring the appointment forward.'

'That's what I thought, but he says he can manage until then. He says it might just go away by itself. He doesn't want to bother the doctor.'

'That's what the doctor is there for,' I say firmly.

'We've always been taught not to be sick, not to go to the doctor for just any old illness. But now I think I will call him.'

Metastases in the head

[30 August] Dr Liem runs his index finger down the list of names on the computer printout.

'I haven't seen Mr Dekker in the waiting room yet,' he mumbles.

'How is he?' I ask, tense.

'Nasty, nasty,' he sighs. 'He's probably got a recurrence, judging by what he said when he phoned me Friday afternoon. Everything points to it. He had an appointment with the neurologist today. That's standard in this trial. He'll still be there. I assume the neurologist will make a CT scan. If it is a recurrence, then it's happened really fast. Let me see if he's here yet.' Dr Liem strides hurriedly toward the waiting room. A few minutes later Dr Liem returns with Mr and Mrs Dekker and Johan. He is walking slowly now so that Mrs Dekker can keep up. They look shaken. Mrs Dekker looks desperate. Mr Dekker tries to feign high spirits but is not succeeding.

'So, what's the problem?' Dr Liem says in a friendly tone. Mr and Mrs Dekker explain, struggling with the words. Dr Liem listens and nods occasionally as he makes notes on the green form in front of him. Before they had arrived, Dr Liem had written, 'Patient coming in early for check-up. Suspect brain metastases. Consult neurologist.'

'The problem with this kind of tumour is that it can recur,' Dr Liem says when they have finished. I'm anticipating things a bit here, but I want to tell you now what I suspect. Maybe it's nothing, and then we can all be relieved, but it is also possible that the tumour has spread to your brain–'

Mrs Dekker starts to cry quietly.

'And then the question is, What do we do next?

They all look tensely at Dr Liem, who taps his pen on the green form on his desk.

'There are possibilities,' Dr Liem says. 'Did you have a lot of trouble with the previous course of treatment?'

'Absolutely not,' Mr Dekker says immediately.

'Well, the treatment I have in mind will be even less troublesome and there'll be less side-effects.'

Mr Dekker nods.

'Will he have to be admitted again?' Mrs Dekker asks.

'No,' Dr Liem answers. 'It would all go through the outpatient clinic. You would come three times in the first week, on Monday, Wednesday and Friday. Then you have three weeks off. Then another three doses of medication.' He draws a time schedule as he talks. 'But I need to find out exactly what is wrong first,' he continues. 'I'll make an appointment for you for Friday. By then we should know more and we can draw up a plan. It all depends on the result of the scan. If they make the scan tomorrow then you must call me, because we can then bring our appointment forward to Wednesday. The earlier the better.' Dr Liem is clearly in a hurry.

Mr Dekker clears his throat. 'That other doctor, Dr Kooiman, he said that the chemotherapy goes through your whole body. If it had spread to other parts then it should reach it there as well, shouldn't it? So I don't understand how this could happen.'

'That's the bad thing about this kind of tumour,' Dr Liem says. 'It tends to come back again.' He makes an apologetic gesture with his arm.

'That's what the neurologist said as well,' says Mrs Dekker.

'It's good that you acted early and phoned us,' Dr Liem compliments them. That gives us more opportunity to act fast. That is important with this kind of tumour.'

'Otherwise . . . ? Mr Dekker begins, looking expectantly at Dr Liem.

'Otherwise things could end quite soon,' Dr Liem adds. 'When you first came here we told you that if we don't do anything then you wouldn't be here two or three months later. The same applies now. If the cancer has come back, then the starting point is less favourable than it was then. But let me not anticipate results we haven't received yet. Let's first wait and see what the scan tells us.' Dr Liem gathers all Mr Dekker's papers together and stands up. 'We'll meet on Friday,' he says, as he extends his hand. He then leaves the room.

Mrs Dekker has trouble getting up out of her chair. I put my arm around her and she now starts to cry in earnest. She takes off her glasses and wipes her eyes. 'We hadn't expected this,' she says. I hear muffled cries coming from Mr Dekker. He weeps as he looks at his wife. He cannot bear to see her like this. Johan leans against the door post. He seems unconcerned, but I know him well enough to know that this is affecting him greatly. I nod at him. 'Great that you can give them some support,' I say. He looks shy.

'He brings us to the hospital,' Mrs Dekker says proudly.

Dr Liem returns to the office with the next patient. I suddenly feel ill at ease, standing in the doorway with my arm around Mrs Dekker, holding up Dr Liem's clinic. Dr Liem smiles at me and says nothing.

'We'll be off then,' Mrs Dekker says. I nod. Mr Dekker wants to touch my cheek but miscalculates and his hand shoots past my face. They leave and I take my place next to Dr Liem for the next patient.

More chemotherapy

[3 September, 8:15 am] On Friday morning I walk over to the outpatient clinic. As I pass the X-ray department I see Mr Dekker in a wheelchair in the waiting room. Johan is with him. They have had a bad week, Mr Dekker explains. He is finding it even more difficult to speak than the last time I saw him. I can hardly understand him at all. The news that the cancer had returned had been hard. Dr Liem had phoned yesterday to say that the scan revealed two tumours in the brain. 'He wants to treat me immediately,' Mr Dekker says with a sob. He is wracked with contradictory feelings; he wonders whether it would have made a difference if he had come back to the hospital earlier, while at the same time feeling that he should not go to the doctor unless it is really necessary.

'He's deteriorating every day,' Johan says.

'Johan had to bring two invalids to hospital,' Mr Dekker jokes. 'He almost had to hire a bus.'

Mrs Dekker is in the outpatient waiting room.

'I've already heard the bad news,' I tell her. She is calmer than on Monday; less upset. 'We haven't slept for two nights,' she says. 'Klaas has been seeing his own funeral.' I go and get some coffee and sit down next to her. They had apparently not anticipated that the cancer could come back. The symptoms were so different from the previous ones; it had taken them completely by surprise. If Mr Dekker had been short of breath again then they could have understood, but not this.

'Vera has been to see the GP,' Mrs Dekker says as she stirs her coffee mechanically with a plastic spoon. 'She says we need him. Our relationship with him is so bad that I wouldn't have called him at all. But he came to see us and we have resolved things.'

'Good,' I say. We sit in silence next to each other and drink our coffee.

[6 September] On Monday afternoon I look into the outpatient infusion room. Mr Dekker is sitting in a large aeroplane chair receiving the second infusion in his first course of treatment. He cannot do much more than sit, he tells me. There is less pressure in his head, he says, and he still thinks it is important to retain a sense of humour.

'This morning I told Rietje that I'm like someone in a slapstick film who can't do anything properly. I fall down, I can't shave myself properly. I can't do anything.'

[8 September] Mr Dekker receives his third course on Wednesday morning. Dr Liem says that he has to lecture on Thursday morning and asks Mr Dekker if he could come and tell his story. Of course he will be there, even if it is the last thing he does. His obedience touches me.

'You've done so much for us,' he says gratefully. 'I'm happy to do something for you in return,' he says.

Recurrence: counselling and emotions

In the period of remission after the first-line chemotherapy rest and recuperation are central. Patients have deteriorated physically during the treatment; most feel worse than they did at the time of diagnosis. The number of hospital visits has drastically reduced and patients only call in for a check-up once every six weeks. They generally try to build up their strength at home. The feeling is, 'The cancer has gone, but I'm not back to normal yet'. Patients and their relatives try to regain some sort of physical and mental equilibrium.

Mr Dekker's recurrence is unexpected. The symptoms are completely different from those at the start of his illness and it is difficult for him and his relatives to accept them as signs of the recurring cancer. They also had not counted on the cancer recurring. Mr Dekker was the first in his 'group' to have brain metastases. When fellow patients later showed similar symptoms they were better prepared because they had seen the development of Mr Dekker's illness.

During the discussion with the doctor during what I will call the second bad news interview, the doctor also informs the patient of his condition in stages. First Dr Liem tells Mr Dekker of his suspicions, thus preparing him for what is to come. The tests, in this case a CT scan, then prove these suspicions. In anticipation of the scan results the doctor tells the patient that if there was a recurrence then it would be possible to treat it. As in the case of the first diagnosis, the aggressive nature of the tumour means that there is no time to lose. In the second bad news interview the doctor is more active in informing the patient about the short-term prognosis.

After the first bad news interview and subsequent treatment patients and their relatives have had to learn to live with the illness. During the period of remission the bad news recedes into the background and the social environment adjusts to the patient's reduced physical competence. The recurrence is a disruption of this new equilibrium. In the second bad news interview patients and their families are once again suddenly confronted by mortality and this fills them with despair and disappointment that, they say, is more intense than after the initial diagnosis. They have struggled hard to get better and now they realize that this has been in vain. The outcome of therapy had not been what they had hoped for, that they had secretly assumed: cure. There is also incomprehension. How is it possible that the cancer has come back in the brain when the chemotherapy was supposed to spread through the whole body?

Mr Wiersema

[8 September] After not having seen them for two months I spot Mr and Mrs Wiersema in the waiting room. They wave and I go across the room and sit next to them. He looks well and they say that things are going well. They have not been to the hospital for six weeks. Mr Wiersema soon turns the conversation toward his fellow-patients.

'Things have gone wrong with Dekker,' he says.

'We phone regularly,' Mrs Wiersema says. 'She said, "We always phone when we have good news, now I'm phoning with bad news."'

Later, when I pass the infusion room I hear talking and laughter. Four men are receiving chemotherapy; one of them is Mr Dekker. Mrs Dekker is next to him, drinking a cup of coffee. The nurse Mark van Rossum jokes with the patients as he adjusts the equipment. Mrs Dekker tells me that things are improving. She tells me that when things had looked extremely bleak the previous week they had experienced an emotionally intense time together. Mr Dekker nods.

'Guess who I just saw in the waiting room,' I say.

'Who?'

'Mr Wiersema.'

'Really?' Mr Dekker says. 'I need to see him. Can you tell him I'm here?'

I go and fetch Mr and Mrs Wiersema and there is a warm reunion.

Later Mr and Mrs Wiersema sit tensely in Dr Liem's office as he scans the X-rays. He takes the old X-rays from an envelope and compares them.

'Terrific,' he exclaims as he turns to the Wiersemas. 'It's a complete remission. Here, let me show you. There you see the lesion.' He points to a white patch on one of the X-rays. 'That's what it looked like halfway through the treatment. You can see the tumour has already reduced by half. And now here, on the most recent X-ray you see nothing at all. Your lungs are completely clear.' He looks cheerfully at Mr Wiersema, who gets up to take a closer look at the X-rays.

'Yes,' he says. 'Can't see anything on this last one. Look, Hanneke.' Mrs Wiersema nods, happy.

'So it looks good?' he says, requesting confirmation from Dr Liem.

Dr Liem nods. 'Very good.'

'But with Dekker things aren't so good?' Mr Wiersema says.

Dr Liem shrugs noncommittally. He does not talk about other patients.

'I couldn't sleep thinking about him,' Mr Wiersema insists.

'Mr Dekker is a *very* different case,' Dr Liem says carefully. 'Patients don't all respond in the same way to therapy.'

Mr Wiersema nods. 'I wasn't looking forward to coming here today,' he says to me.

'Did it keep you awake last night?' I ask.

'Mrs Wiersema nods fiercely. Earlier she had told me that he was already nervous a week before his check-up appointments.

'Yes,' Mr Wiersema says. Then turning to Dr Liem, 'So things look good, do they?'

'Mr Wiersema, if I didn't already know your case, I wouldn't even be able to tell from this X-ray where the lesion was. I can't see a thing. Of course, it's still possible that the odd cell has remained behind somewhere, and that we can't see it on the X-ray. That's always a possibility. We'll have to wait and see.'

Mr Wiersema becomes playful and wants me to measure his blood pressure.

'There's still a neurological examination,' Dr Liem says. 'We want to look at the side effects of the chemotherapy. I don't expect much to come out of that. The chemotherapy that you had sometimes affects the nerve endings. Gives you a numb sensation in your fingertips. You shouldn't worry though, it's just a side effect. You only need to come back and see me in six weeks.'

The other patient's recurrence

Mr Wiersema was doing fine. He was (still) in the phase of rest and remission. From the doctor he has heard only good news. His lungs were 'clear'. Doctors qualified messages such as, 'I can't see anything on the X-ray,' with a veiled warning like, 'It's still possible that the odd cell has remained behind somewhere'. Patients do not interpret these words as a warning, however, possibly because they do not want to hear bad news. Moreover, it is difficult for a lay person to interpret the disappearance of worrying patches on the X-ray as anything other than positive.

I referred to a veiled warning. Less charitably I could describe the doctor's words simply as inaccurate. The doctor knows that it is not only possible that the odd cell has remained behind but quite certain. In cases like that of Mr Wiersema with small-cell lung carcinoma extended disease it is certain that the tumour will return.

But something has changed. In earlier meetings the doctor's positive messages satisfied Mr Wiersema. Later on this was only partially the case. Mr Dekker's recurrence has made him think more critically about his own future. The realization that his fellow patient is vulnerable has made Mr Wiersema think about his own vulnerability. Glaser and Strauss (1965) call this 'rehearsal'. Patients observe each other fearfully, looking for signs of what is in store for themselves.

Dr Liem's reaction to Mr Wiersema's anxiety is typical of the way doctors talk to patients in remission about other patients with a recurrence. Dr Liem first tries to change the subject. When the patient insists he individualizes Mr Dekker as 'a very different case'. By diverting attention from Mr Dekker the doctor tries to reduce Mr Wiersema's anxiety (de Swaan 1985; Costain Schou 1993).

The lecture

[9 September] I sit next to Dorien Meulman in the lecture theatre listening to Dr Liem expound on the small-cell lung carcinoma. There are about 150 students attending the lecture.

'I would now like to introduce you to Mr Dekker,' Dr Liem says, introducing his patient. Johan pushes Mr Dekker down the aisle to the front of the theatre. Dr Liem takes the microphone and sits next to Mr Dekker.

'Mr Dekker, could you tell us what the complaints were that first made you consult a doctor?'

'I was terribly tired,' Mr Dekker answers.

'When was this?'

'Last December.'

'Please continue.'

'I was gradually getting more tired. I couldn't disguise it any more. There was a reason for wanting to hide it. My wife is disabled and I didn't want to burden her.'

'Have you ever smoked?'

'Yes, a lot.' Mr Dekker nods. 'But I stopped immediately in December.'

'Then you received treatment?'

'Yes, once they knew what I had I was given chemotherapy within the week.'

'Did you have any complaints during treatment?'

'No, almost nothing. I wasn't nauseous or anything. I did cough up some blood once.'

Dr Liem takes the microphone and addresses the audience. 'The patient had greatly improved after six courses of treatment. But the tumour hadn't disappeared completely.'

I look at Mr Dekker, down in the front of the lecture theatre. I remember him telling me that the cancer has disappeared completely and I have the feeling that perhaps he has now just realized what the situation really is.

'A few weeks after the chemotherapy things started to get worse,' Dr Liem continues. 'Mr Dekker, what happened exactly?'

'I started to have problems walking, I couldn't see properly, I couldn't talk properly, I kept choking when I swallowed. After a couple of weeks I could hardly do anything. I thought I'd had a stroke or something.'

Dr Liem addresses the students. 'If this patient reported to you with these symptoms, what would you suspect was wrong with him?'

There is silence. No one dares to say anything, even though Dr Liem has already described the course of the illness in his introduction. (Later he tells me that some of the students complained that they thought it unethical to discuss patients like that in their presence.) Eventually someone dares to suggest a possible recurrence.

'Very good,' Dr Liem says. 'Mr Dekker did indeed have a recurrence. We also tackled that with chemotherapy and now things are a lot better.' He turns to his patient.

'I could hardly talk at all last week,' Mr Dekker confirms. And now I can. I can also walk. I'm in a wheelchair now, but that's only because it's so far from the car to here.'

Loyalty toward the doctor

I have described Mr Dekker's role in Dr Liem's lecture because it expresses so clearly patients' loyalty toward the doctor who is treating them. Mr Dekker is almost thankful when Dr Liem asks him to participate in the lecture. At last he is able to reciprocate, to do something for the doctor who takes care of him and who is always ready to help him.

Mr Dekker agrees to participate at a time when he is under a lot of physical and emotional stress. He and his family are having a hard time. The brain metastases make it difficult for him to talk and he is in a wheelchair. His very appearance defines him as the patient, the person with physical defects. I can imagine that at this moment, when he has hardly had time to get used to these new physical defects, he finds it humiliating to talk about his illness in such a public setting. He never told me this, but I could not avoid that impression when I saw him, before all those students, trying his best to appear normal.

I found that patients were often surprisingly loyal toward their doctors. I cannot remember patients ever complaining about the continual interruptions of consultations and difficult conversations by the bleeping of the doctor's pager. It was only very occasionally that a patient became angry about the sometimes very long time spent in waiting rooms. Doctors did not need to insist when they needed a patient to collaborate in a clinical trial. Patients always complied and were often keen to participate in trials of new medication, often in the hope that it might be just that much better than existing therapy. The patients who were critical were often more highly educated than average. Occasionally adult children of less educated patients might complain about long waiting times of a poorly prepared consultation.

The nurse Mark van Rossum pointed to this loyalty (Chapter 2). He described the patient's need to 'accommodate' the doctor and not disappoint. I think that Mark was right in this interpretation. I sometimes had the impression that patients thought they were privileged that doctors devoted their valuable time to them (de Swaan 1985). This is rather ironic, given that it is the patient's time that is the scarce resource (The et al. 1996). It seemed as though patients tried to cause as little trouble as possible and to be as pleasant as they could, because they thought that this would be better for the treatment.

I have already discussed the patients' desire to 'do something' for the doctor. What I said there is applicable in this context as well. Patients desire to be treated more than anything else and will do anything to achieve this. For them, treatment has priority over everything else. The doctor makes the decisions and directs treatment. The only thing left for patients to do is to cooperate, and they do that by not complaining, by down playing the side effects when talking to the doctor and by emphasizing trust in the doctor. Trust in the doctor is central and patients surrender themselves to the treatment. The dominant view is: doctor knows best and even if we do not understand what he is doing he will have his reasons. Distrust and criticism in such a relationship would be out of place.

Many patients feel that they have no right to occupy doctors' time with non-medical issues. This is partly because doctors have taught them this. As I have mentioned several times, doctors consider their task to be medical. In the discussion in which he told Ronald Westra that Brigit would soon die, Dr Veerman said quite explicitly that he was not the right person to discuss psychosocial support. In the following chapters I give examples in which 'having no right to non-medical attention' play a role. In the next chapter Mr Dekker leads his sobbing wife out of the doctor's office because he does not want to keep him from his work. And in Chapter 10, Mr Mulder's daughter apologizes for talking about her family at the end of a consultation in which the doctor has told her that they can do nothing more for her father and that he will soon die.

Mr Dekker feels unwell again

[20 September] Mr Dekker's second course of therapy is delayed a week because his blood has not yet recovered. When he does receive his treatment he does not cope well. He is dizzy, has double vision and is unable to talk properly.

'Klaas is down,' Mrs Dekker says.

'I'm worried that the treatment isn't working,' Mr Dekker says. 'Is that pos-sible?' he asks me, only to answer his own question before I have a chance to speak. 'Ach, you wouldn't know that, would you?'

Mrs Dekker says that the nights are the worst. He is scared that he will wake up and be unable to express himself. When she wakes up the first thing she does is to check whether he is okay. The news that the cancer had returned was a hard blow, more difficult to cope with than the initial diagnosis. 'We fought so hard. We thought we were winning. And now this.' They are disappointed.

Later Dr Heller reassures them. 'We're just going to persevere,' he says after hearing their fears. 'The treatment has to be given the chance to do its work. After this course we'll make a scan of your head to see if it's had any effect.

[1 October] Mr Dekker receives the last infusion in his second course of treat-ment. The scan was made the previous day.

'I don't think that the treatment is working,' he says. His stepdaughter is sitting on a stool next to the aeroplane seat in which he receives his treatment. 'If it was then there should have been some effect earlier, shouldn't there? I'm still seeing things double. It's not getting better. But I want to keep the humour in.' I nod and feel a lump in my throat.

'If I have to kick the bucket then I want to do so laughing,' he says. He says the words with difficulty. 'They have to have a good memory of me. That's life. Crying and emotion will get us nowhere.'

I steal a glance at Vera. The tears are streaming down her cheeks. It is the first time I have heard him talking about dying.

[3 October] Mr Bokjes asks Dr Liem whether he can go on holiday. Dr Liem says it is okay, but without conviction. He looks at the X-ray for a long time. 'There are some white dashes here,' he says. 'We'll have to wait and see how they develop. If you come back in two weeks then we can discuss further. And you can tell me about your holiday.' When they have left he tells me that he is almost certain that Mr Bokjes has a recurrence. Usually he tells the patient of his suspicions. In the case of Mr Bokjes he wants to wait until he is certain. 'Other-wise they're likely to panic,' he explains. 'Mr Bokjes didn't respond well to the chemotherapy. It made him feel ill, and I'm not sure whether we should treat him again. It's too much for him.'

Mr Dekker's progression

[8 October] Mr and Mrs Dekker come to see Dr Heller to discuss the results of the scan. He has already informed them that the scan had revealed progression. What were the options? This depends on Mr Dekker's condition. Radiotherapy is probably the best option.

'How are things?' Dr Heller asks when they are seated opposite him.

'Perfect,' Mr Dekker answers. 'No complaints at all. I feel on top of the world.' He does look better than he did at the previous appointment.

'Klaas is exaggerating,' Mrs Dekker says.

'What do you do during the day?' Dr Heller asks.

'Upholstery. I've got a new hobby. I'm doing a chair for my brother.' ('No, I've gone off that,' he says later when I ask him about the soldiers. 'He can't manage,' his wife adds.)

Mrs Dekker is worried. 'He's pretending to be much better than he is. How are the X-rays?'

'To be honest you look better than the X-rays,' Dr Heller says. 'The treatment isn't working.'

The colour drains from Mr Dekker's face. 'It's better than the other way round,' he says.

'We had anticipated as much,' Mrs Dekker says quietly.

'I'm sorry,' Dr Heller says. He phones the neurologist to discuss treatment. They agree to give him *dexametason* for a few days and then radiotherapy.

'Next week you'll get a call for the radiotherapy. Then in four weeks you come here again for a check-up.'

At the reception desk Mr Dekker is waiting for his hospital pass. 'Koster came to visit us the other day,' he says. 'He was in bad shape. He was shaking so much he couldn't hold his cup of coffee. I saw Wiersema a couple of weeks ago and he's only just managing. Let's be honest, sooner or later we'll all get the blow. That's how I see it, we'll all go sooner or later.'

'Yes,' I say, testing how far he will go. 'We all have to go sometime.'

'No,' he corrects me. 'That's not what I mean. I mean that Wiersema, Bokjes, Koster and me, we are all going to die of *this disease*.'

[14 October] Mr and Mrs Dekker are now going to the radiotherapy department and I lose sight of them. After two weeks I phone them at home to find out how they are doing.

'Worse,' Mr Dekker says. 'I'm having more difficulty with walking and talking. Rietje wants to talk to you.'

'Klaas in emotional,' she says. She says he feels pressure in his head and that his personality is changing.

Mr Dekker becomes aware

Mr Dekker has changed. The eruptions of euphoria with Mr Wiersema seem very distant. I notice that he is increasingly thinking about death. I suspect that he is becoming aware not only that his illness is fatal but also that it will be rapidly fatal. I do not dare discuss it with him. I am not sure whether this is the right moment and I am uncertain as to how to broach the topic. I am afraid to hurt him, but at the same time I find myself cowardly in discussing superficial topics when there are obviously more pressing issues on Mr Dekker's mind. I comfort myself by thinking that I should be studying the process that Mr Dekker is going through and should therefore not be influencing it unduly. Then, unexpectedly, at the outpatient reception desk, Mr Dekker suddenly shares this realization with me, 'We are all going to die of this disease'.

During their illness patients gradually become conscious of what is happening. Various people play a role in this. This not only applies to Mr Dekker but to all the patients I studied. The way in which patients are informed is the first factor. The blow is a hard one. In the bad news interview the patient is given a death sentence. Subsequently, during therapy, the long-term prognosis, fatal outcome of the illness, is not mentioned by the doctor. Indeed, the discourse during this period is exclusively concerned with the short term, and is generally favourable. Information is provided passively, only in response to requests by the patient.

It was only when the illness recurred that Dr Liem spoke of it as being incurable. During the lecture Mr Dekker heard a description of the course of the illness, this time in more neutral terms. While I watched Mr Dekker listening to the more abstract details of his illness I had the impression that something changed. I had the impression that he suddenly realized what the truth of his situation was. It seemed as though something in him snapped. He did not hear anything new, it was the same information but couched in different terms. That this information had an effect on him is supported by his unusual behaviour after the lecture. He went straight home, rather than lingering for a drink and a chat as he was wont to do. Repetition of the bad news contributes to the patient's realization of impending death. Different terminology, setting and perhaps audience as well, contribute to this process.

It is also important that during their illness patients feel themselves deteriorating physically. The first-line chemotherapy drains them physically. Then the recurrence is usually accompanied by more complaints than the initial diagnosis. In the period of the initial diagnosis the doctor's words do not coincide with the patient's illness experience. It is difficult for patients to realize that they are fatally ill.[1] In the phase in which patients develop a recurrence, their experience of their illness and the words of the doctor do coincide. Because patients now feel ill, what the doctor says sounds different from what he said during the first bad news interview. It sounds much less incredible that they are going to be abandoned by their bodies. Various patients and their partners told me that in this phase of deterioration they

---

1 Mr Dekker is not a good example here as he did suspect, before the diagnosis, that he was going to die. However, in this section I am discussing the general line rather than individual patients.

realized what the doctor had meant when he spoke of 'not getting better'. They had previously heard what he said, but they had not grasped its full meaning. It is a well-known phenomenon. You can tell children not to play with matches otherwise they will get burned, but they only grasp the full meaning of 'getting burned' when they burn themselves. The meaning is only fully brought home by the experience.

The news that the second-line therapy was not having an effect was disappointing for Mr Dekker, but it was not unexpected. He felt his physical condition deteriorate and so his body had prepared him for the news. Patients who have reached the stage that Mr Dekker was in, who are soon to die, often seem to realize that they are approaching the end. Mr Dekker had a feeling for what was to come. The fact that he had the example of Brigit Westra, a fellow patient who was ahead of him in the illness trajectory, also played a role.

The final factor I want to mention here is time. Patients need time to develop towards the realization of death. The realization of approaching death is a gradual process; it can be guided but not forced (The et al. 1996). When Dr Liem tells Mr Dekker about the recurrence and his prognosis he is emotionally receptive to the realization that he is going to die.

Mr Bokjes' recurrence

[15 October] 'And the next patient is Mr Bokjes,' Dr Liem says. 'Let me go and get him.' A few minutes later he returns followed by Mr and Mrs Bokjes. Dr Liem raises his eyebrows when he catches my eye. 'Things are not looking good,' he whispers to me as he passes. Mr Bokjes's face is swollen and red. It looks as though it might explode at any minute. When Dr Liem asks him how he feels Mr Bokjes launches into a nervous exposition.

'I'm at home, washing the dishes, see, and I see my reflection in the window, and I think to myself, you're looking really strange today. Where has that come from? So I tell her, I say, we have to phone the doctor. But the doctor says we need to discuss it with the hospital. Doctor, I keep crying. I just spontaneously start to cry,' he says, wiping his eyes.

'There are glands that are pressing on blood vessels,' Dr Liem explains. 'That's why your face is so swollen. He explains that this is a consequence of the recurring tumour. 'You'll have to undergo another course of treatment. That will improve things. I want to initiate that today.'

'Oh oh oh,' Mrs Bokjes sighs.

'Is it going to make me nauseous? Mr Bokjes sobs. 'We'll have to go through that whole circus with the food again.'

'This treatment is not as strong as the previous one,' Dr Liem reassures him. 'You will receive the first course today, and then the next two on Friday and Monday.'

'No, I can't make it on Friday. I have to go to the doctor for my back,' Mr Bokjes protests.

'And on Monday I've got a birthday party,' Mrs Bokjes remembers.

'This is more important,' Dr Liem insists firmly. 'This is *much* more important than anything else.'

'Yes yes of course,' says Mrs Bokjes, her hand in front of her mouth. 'I don't want to lose my husband, doctor. Please, no.'

Shortly after Mr and Mrs Bokjes leave arm in arm, Mr Bokjes sobbing. Dr Liem phones their GP. 'She was surprised,' he says to me when he has hung up. 'She hadn't realized.'

'I think that Mrs Bokjes does realize what's going on,' I say. 'She said she didn't want to lose her husband. She realizes what the treatment is about.'

'She doesn't understand at all,' Dr Liem says. 'But she is going to lose him. He's going to die. He's got extended disease, which means that even with the chemotherapy the survival time is less than two years.' He sighs. 'I have the feeling that even though I try to explain things as simply as possible to them they still don't understand.'

The doctor leads through the chaos

I have described the discussions between Dr Liem and Mr Bokjes to illustrate a variation in the pattern of information provision. The way in which the doctor provides information varies from one patient to another. As in the case of Mr Dekker, Mr and Mrs Bokjes did not recognize his symptoms as signalling a recurrence of the same disease. The swelling of Mr Bokjes' face took them completely by surprise and it frightens them. They are emotional, panicky and confused. They do not have the situation under control. Everything seems to them to be of equal importance: the swollen face, the birthday party, the recurrence, the treatment. Their story resembles that of Mrs Heuvel in Chapter 1: a chaos narrative (Frank 1995).

Dr Liem is reluctant to treat Mr Bokjes again because he is unsure whether the patient will be able to cope with another course of treatment. He had already seen how Mr Bokjes had difficulty coping with the first-line chemotherapy, how reluctant he was to be admitted to hospital, how he spent large parts of the day crying in bed. Mr Bokjes also had a lot of side effects, particularly nausea. The nausea was also partly a result of nerves. 'Mr Bokjes becomes nauseous when he enters my office,' Dr Heller once told me. It was these considerations that made Dr Liem decide not to interrupt Mr Bokjes's happy holiday plans with news of the recurrence.

When Mr Bokjes reports experiencing symptoms of the tumour during the next consultation, Dr Liem decides to treat him. This time he takes complete control. Instead of discussing the options with the patient, he tells him that he is going to treat him, ignoring complaints about side effects and other appointments. One of the reasons for this sudden decision to treat was the appearance of the vena cava superior syndrome. The case of Mr Bokjes illustrates how doctors adjust their information and offer of treatment to each patient.

'In practice the doctor decides'

Once a week doctors attend a 'discharge meeting' during which they discuss all the patients who have been discharged from hospital during that week.

'We had Mrs Fisher-Rijn, admitted for a course of VIMP [Vincristine Ifosfamide Mesna Carboplatin] chemotherapy,' says Jack Molenaar, a new junior doctor. 'She is a 63-year-old lady with a small-cell lung carcinoma with brain metastases. Previous treatment was ineffective and so she has been given VIMP.'

'That's normal in the case of small-cell lung carcinoma,' Ronald Veerman corrects him. 'It often happens that the treatment has an effect but that the tumour later recurs. So you can't say that the treatment was ineffective.'

As we walk back to our offices after the meeting, Ronald Veerman tells me that statements like that really irritate him. 'I didn't say much because he's new,' he says. 'Of course I know that I can't cure them, but we can't cure people with COPD either, but that doesn't stop us from giving them prednison. You don't tell them you're not going to give them anything because you can't cure them. What alternative do they have? Death. That's not an acceptable alternative for anyone. With chemotherapy, someone like that might live for another couple of years. You can't deprive them of that.'

We have reached my office and as we linger in the doorway I ask him to come in for a cup of coffee. He takes a seat in one of the old chairs. 'I often see that after the first-line chemotherapy,' he continues. 'After they have passed the first acute stage and are feeling a bit better, patients start to think about what they want. They're already weighing up the options before the recurrence. I can see that they are thinking about these issues when they come in for their check-ups. I have the impression that patients are more convinced of the necessity of second-line therapy than they are of first-line therapy.'

'I have the impression that patients become despondent when they have to repeat the whole procedure,' I say. 'They wonder, "Why should I bother when it's going to come back anyway?" They realize that they are not going to be cured.'

'Yes,' the doctor nods. 'There is a terrible disappointment. But I go a step further. The disappointment is there. I tell them, then I ask them to come back a week later when they have had time to calm down and think. I've never once had the experience that they come back and tell me they don't want to go through with the next course. Of course, the way in which I provide the information probably has a big influence on the patient. My experience is that if patients detect any sign of doubt in the doctor then they respond to it. If patients are unsure what to do and I say I don't think it is a good idea, then they definitely wouldn't agree to treatment.'

'You have power,' I say.

'Exactly, that's what I'm saying. In practice it's the doctor who decides what happens.'

'But the advantage of treatment is that you live for a year and a half longer,' I say. 'I can imagine that a year and a half is more important for some than for others. And non-medical factors also play a role: existential questions, financial matters, personal issues that need completing, subjective factors. It seems to me that such non-medical factors make it more difficult for the doctor. You say the doctor decides. Do you also take these factors into account?'

'Yes, certainly. I once had a patient who had very clear ideas on those issues. He had a tumour, was treated and went home. Six months later the tumour returned and he refused further treatment. He had thought about it. He didn't have a family. After the first course of treatment he had gone back to his work and his social life, but with the second tumour he decided that he had had a good life and that it was time to go. He was consistent in this opinion during two discussions I had with him and I accepted. I don't have a problem with that.'

'Okay, that patient raised the matter himself. But do you take the initiative in asking about these things?'

'If it's someone from East Groningen then I do,' he answers with a smile.[2] That might sound strange, but the people from this region are very closed. You know that they are going to tell you that everything is fine, even though it isn't. In those cases I claim the opposite in order to try and get a better picture. I also think it's important that they come with someone else. Then I can get information from different sources. It gives me a feeling for the situation and helps in making decisions. I think these are important issues. You're treating a person, not a small-cell lung carcinoma. It's the person who should benefit.'

'Would it help patients in making those difficult decisions if people other than doctors were involved?'

'We need to ask ourselves whether we doctors should be the ones deciding. There are also others, like the psychologist or the pastor. We need to ask whether we should be more intensively involved, or whether we should involve more people in order to reach a better considered verdict. I personally think that would be better, but it isn't economically feasible.

'As doctor you can point to certain issues, but the patient also has to contribute. You should make difficult decisions like that together with the patient. In practice a lot of patients don't say anything at all; they want the doctor to decide. Then you get the responsibility that you're trying to share played back to you, and sooner or later a decision has to be made. There have been occasions when I've found it very difficult; so difficult that I wasn't sure what to decide. So

---

2 A rural farming area in the far north-east of the Netherlands.

I consulted the GP. But in the final instance I think that patients should decide themselves. If someone is 90 and they want to live, then I have the duty to do all in my power to help them. Age is irrelevant to the decision and you can't discriminate on the basis of age. Though you can discriminate on medical grounds: how good is their heart, their kidneys. Those are traditional selection criteria.'

On choosing therapy once again

Dr Veerman describes the pattern of choice for second-line chemotherapy. What it boils down to is that doctors always offer therapy unless it is medically contra-indicated. Sometimes doctors annotate the decision and offer some resistance, as Ronald Veerman describes in the case of Mr Rulofs. But if patients want therapy then they get it. In the case of Mr Bokjes we see how Dr Liem doubted on partly non-medical grounds whether he would offer the patient therapy. I saw this doubt more often, but it never resulted in the doctor not offering the treatment option.

Ronald Veerman is right when he says that patients never refuse second-line chemotherapy. There were, however, differences compared to first-line therapy. The most striking was that patients openly discussed the advantages and disadvantages. After initially receiving their diagnosis patients hardly thought about treatment options. They felt as though they had their backs to the wall and that there was no real choice. They ignored side effects and acceptance of treatment was obvious.

When they reach second-line therapy patients have already undergone therapy and thus experienced what they are choosing. The memories of side effects are still fresh in their memory. Moreover, the therapy has not had the desired effect. They are not, as they initially hoped, cured. The cancer has come back and with it the realization that the illness is incurable and treatment intended merely to extend life. They begin to wonder whether therapy is worth it if the cancer is going to keep coming back anyway.

On the other hand, these considerations motivate some patients to accept therapy. Because the tumour has returned, they are even more fearful of what the future has to offer. There is a general tendency to express doubts and fears more clearly. These doubts did not lead to any of the patients in my study refusing second-line chemotherapy.

8 Declining optimism

'You have to reap the benefits of treatment *now*'

[20 October] Mr Wiersema comes for a check-up. He is in the waiting room with his wife. She removes her handbag from the seat next to her and I sit down. Things are going well and he has been doing some painting and decorating at home. When Mr Wiersema goes in for his blood test, Mrs Wiersema stays in the waiting room with me.

'Joop has spoken to Klaas Dekker,' she tells me. 'I heard him ask about the precise symptoms of a tumour in the brain. He projects everything onto himself. Every little pain leads to the fear that it's the cancer that's come back. I try to reassure him. I tell him he hasn't got the swollen glands like Klaas Dekker had. Joop had a tumour in his liver, but that disappeared after treatment.'

The conversation was interrupted by the arrival of Mr Koster and his daughter. Mr Koster says that his tumour has completely disappeared as a result of therapy but that it has affected him. 'He's become a vegetable,' his daughter adds. Mr Wiersema receives good news from the doctor. There are no signs of metastases. The only problem is high blood pressure, for which he receives medication. Next check-up in six weeks.

Mr Koster tells Dr Liem that it is taking a long time for him to feel better and that he is looking forward to better times. The doctor explains that Mr Koster has a very aggressive form of cancer. 'The advantage of treatment,' Dr Liem explains, 'is that it's made it possible for you to still be here now.' The patient nods. 'The disadvantage of the treatment is the side effects,' Dr Liem continues. 'And the tumour can come back, though we hope that it will keep away as long as possible.' The patient nods again. 'The thing is, you have to reap the benefits of the treatment *now*. You have to enjoy life now, and do the things you enjoy.'

At the end of the meeting they shake hands and Mr Koster says, 'Doctor, I have this problem. I don't know whether I should sell the farm or not. Something inside me says I should keep it on.'

'If you can get a good price for it then I would sell,' Dr Liem says resolutely.

'Are they telling me everything?'

[27 October] In the morning I am in Dr Liem's office, where I receive a phone call from Mrs Dekker. She says she has been trying to reach me since yesterday. She is upset. Yesterday she had a terrible discussion with one of the radiologists, who had been cold and insensitive, she said. 'I've just got so many questions,' she says. 'But nobody is answering them. I've lost my trust in the doctors in the hospital. Are they telling me everything? Is he going to get better or isn't he? I don't dare to ask the doctor again.'

I look across the table at Dr Liem hurriedly sorting through his papers as he prepares for the morning's outpatient clinic, unaware that he is the subject of discussion. Should I pass the phone over to him? I wonder. Would that help Mrs Dekker? How would the doctor construe my contact with his patients? Would that have repercussions for my study? I am a guest in the hospital after all. I am allowed to watch, but must be careful not to disturb the natural course of events.

'That's really unpleasant,' I say. 'I can imagine you're worried, but I'm sorry, I don't know either. As you know, I'm not a doctor.' I try to find a way out for myself. 'I'll call you back after the clinic,' I say.

When we speak later she has calmed down. Klaas has changed, she says. He has become another man. She wants to know whether it is due to his diabetes or to the cancer. Also, he has only had ten sessions of radiotherapy, while others get 30. She wants to know why. 'Have they written him off, Anne-Mei?' she asks. This was the pressing question that she had put to the radiologist, but he had told her to ask the lung specialist. 'I can understand that the doctors are just doing their job and see things differently. But I only have one husband,' she says. She does not want to burden the stepchildren with her worries. 'You're not a doctor,' she says. 'But I have to talk to somebody. I hope you don't mind.' I advise her to make an appointment to discuss the matter with Dr Liem.

[28 October] Mrs Dekker is calmer on the phone. Her problems have not been solved, but she feels more able to face them now. It is difficult for her to see her husband, once so strong, in this condition. He is now in a rehabilitation centre because of his diabetes. 'He's crying all the time,' she says. 'He's terribly emotional. I discuss the things I want to ask the doctor the evening before and he agrees, but when we get there he keeps interrupting me and saying we shouldn't anticipate events. He's scared.' Mrs Wiersema has phoned, and that sympathy had helped.

Mr Wiersema's numbness

[3 November] Two weeks after our last meeting I see Mr and Mrs Wiersema in the waiting room. Surprised, I walk over to them.

'Not so long ago, is it?' says Mr Wiersema without looking at me.

'It's not good,' says Mrs Wiersema, gesturing toward her husband.

'I've gone numb in my right ear,' he says. 'And I keep feeling cold. We phoned Dr Heller and he said we should come in today. Maybe we'll have to see the neurologist.' He looks scared, avoids eye contact with me.

'We could just ignore it, but that wouldn't help,' his wife says.

'Ach ach,' he says, as though he is talking to himself. 'Things are not good with poor old Dekker.'

'Yes,' she says. 'He's having a hard time. They gave him a new course of chemo, but that didn't help. So now he's had ten doses of radiotherapy. And now his diabetes is playing up as well. I went to visit him in the rehabilitation centre.'

'We always phoned each other,' Mr Wiersema says. 'So we still do that. But things are not going well for Joop. And I didn't sleep at all last night.'

'Don't go comparing yourself to others,' Mrs Wiersema says. 'You know you shouldn't do that, but you go on and do it anyway.'

Dr Heller listens attentively to Mr Wiersema's complaints. When he has finished, Dr Heller asks, 'How's your strength?'

Mr Wiersema rolls up his sleeve. 'Try me,' he says as he plants his elbow on the table and sticks out his hand. Mr Wiersema wins easily with both arms.

'I don't think it's as bad as I initially thought over the phone,' Dr Heller says. I think it's being caused by the pills for the high blood pressure. Your body has to get used to them. It will go away by itself. These symptoms are not side effects of the chemotherapy, and from what I can tell they're not related to the cancer either. Let's keep the appointment that we made last time. If the complaints become worse then you can come in earlier.'

After they have left Dr Heller says to me, 'That's definitely not a recurrence. He beat me easily. That would have been impossible with a recurrence.'

The worry increases

Among patients who have not (yet) developed a recurrence and their families the worry about what the future holds gradually increases. One explanation for this is that during the course of the illness doctors are increasingly open with patients about their illness. Dr Liem tells Mr Koster that the cancer can come back and that he has to reap the benefits of treatment while he can. Doctors also frequently warned patients indirectly of what was to come, as Dr Liem did when he advised Mr Koster to sell his farm.

Another factor that adds to the worry is the confrontation with other patients. It is much easier for Mr Wiersema to interpret these new symptoms than it was for Mr Dekker because he already has the example of Mr Dekker. Even though Dr Liem tries to relieve Mr Wiersema's worry by saying that Mr Dekker's case is 'completely different,' Mr Wiersema is not entirely convinced.

Mrs Dekker has other reasons for worrying. She experiences a discrepancy between two sources of information. On the one hand she hears the doctors saying that her husband is doing fine, while at the same time she sees his condition deteriorate. She realizes that something is wrong and suspects that the doctors are not telling her the whole truth. She feels she is losing control over the situation and this makes her desperate and angry.

Here I need to note that it is not only the doctors who have given Mrs Dekker 'wrong' information, but also her husband himself. Because of her handicap Mrs Dekker did not always accompany her husband to his outpatient clinic appointments. As a result much of her information has been derived from what he has told her. I have described above how Mr Dekker always asked the doctor at the end of each consultation whether he was satisfied. The doctor always answered in the affirmative and Mr Dekker passed this on to his wife when he got home.

Mrs Dekker has now started to ask the doctors directly what her husband's situation is. She asked the radiotherapist, who told her to see the doctor in charge of her husband's treatment. Just like the nurses, doctors also refer patients' questions to the doctor responsible. This 'passing the buck' makes Mrs Dekker even more worried. If there were nothing to worry about then surely the radiotherapist would have said so. She could ask Dr Liem but she does not dare to. So she asks me. Perhaps she asks me because he is distant and unapproachable. But perhaps she asks me because she knows that I cannot tell her the truth.[1]

Mrs Dekker is starting to realize that her husband is going to die. She is going through a process of development similar to that of Mr Dekker, but she is in an earlier phase. In most cases the process was not synchronic in both partners. This is partly because patients are more aware of their own physical deterioration. But it is also due to them wanting to hide the real situation in order to protect their loved ones from the hard truth.

Dr Racz

[5 November] Mr and Mrs Dekker and Vera are in the waiting room. 'I phoned Dr Liem and made an appointment,' Mrs Dekker says when she sees me.

---

1 See The (1997a, 1998) on euthanasia requests. Patients often direct requests for euthanasia to nurses rather than doctors. The shorter social and physical distance between nurses and patients is part of the reason for this, but it is also possible that different levels of responsibility also play a role. Discussing euthanasia with nurses does not have any practical consequence because nurses are not qualified to decide on such matters.

'Are you tense?' I ask.

'Yes, but I have to know what the situation is.'

When I go into the office I see Dr Liem and Ilona Racz, a junior doctor, preparing for the outpatient clinic. 'Then there is Mr Dekker,' Dr Liem is saying. 'You have to see him. A man who's had *cisplatinum-etoposide*. A recurrence. We tried *tenoposide* but it had no effect. You don't have to do anything, it's just a check-up. Make a new appointment for six weeks.' Ilona Racz nods.

'Then the next patient,' Dr Liem continues. I want to intervene because I know how important this appointment is for Mrs Dekker. I am surprised that Dr Liem does not seem to realize. But I keep quiet. Ilona Racz is very involved with the patients. She would be the ideal person for this interview. I do not dare say anything. Dr Liem has reached the last patient, the files on his desk are piled high, the waiting room is full and consultations are about to begin. I go into the waiting room to warn Mrs Dekker that they are not going to be seeing Dr Liem. 'But she is good,' I tell them. 'And she listens.' Mrs Dekker is irritated at having to see another doctor, but Mr Dekker simply shrugs.

Back in the office Ilona Racz is looking attentively at Mr Dekker's latest X-rays. 'There's some slight improvement,' she says to me. 'But I think I'll say the situation is stable, otherwise it create expectations. Guido mentioned a recurrence, but I don't see any sign of that.'

'There are brain metastases,' I say.

'Oh, I didn't know that,' she says. She opened Mr Dekkers file and rummages through the papers.

'He's had radiotherapy,' I add.

'Oh, you know him?'

'Yes. Mrs Dekker phoned Guido last week because there were some questions she wanted to ask him.'

'Mmm, so now I have to deal with them. I don't like the way patients keep having to see different doctors. I don't know anything about this patient. Shall I ask Guido to see them? It's probably much better for them.' She looks at me questioningly. I shake my head.

'I think it would be good if you saw them this time,' I say.

'Okay,' she says and walks to the door. 'Let me go and get them.'

The interview with Mrs Dekker

'How are things?' Ilona Racz asks the Dekkers when they are seated opposite her. Vera has remained in the waiting room.

'Better,' Mr Dekker responds immediately. 'Much better.'

'I have a lot of questions for which I never seem to be able to get answers,' says Mrs Dekker emotionally. 'And I find it very unpleasant to have to ask you, because you haven't been involved.'

'Just try and tell me,' Ilona says. 'I'm also a member of this club. I'm represent- ing the other doctors at the moment, so just throw it all at me.' Mrs Dekker looks helplessly at me, as she will continue to do throughout the interview. I nod back encouragingly.

'You say that things look better,' Mrs Dekker says. 'Is that because of the radiotherapy or because of the treatment for his diabetes? I've asked this a number of times, but don't get an answer. I asked the radiotherapist, a horrible woman, but she wouldn't tell me. I'm so uncertain. I can't take it.' She cries and is angry at the same time. Ilona Racz listens patiently and replies that she also has not an answer to that question.

'Are you going to make another scan?' Mrs Dekker asks.

Dr Racz shakes her head. 'Only if there are new complaints.'

'Why do you only do tests when he has complaints? Why don't you check to see whether it's gone? The first time he had chemotherapy they did a scan at the beginning and at the end.'

'Radiotherapy always works. Patients always feel better after radiotherapy. It's much more important to wait and see whether he develops complaints. If so, if he's short of breath or in pain, then we try and do something about it.'

'Have you written him off perhaps?' Mrs Dekker asks in a shrill voice.

'I've tried to explain to her that you can't see the cancer cells on the X-ray but . . .' Mr Dekker begins.

'Dr Kooiman said they were trying to get rid of the tumour,' Mrs Dekker continues, her voice jumping up an octave. But the next thing you know he's coughing up blood. Then he starts talking funny. Then I start doubting.'

Ilona Racz takes her time. 'Your husband has an aggressive tumour,' she explains. That tumour is like a spider that is making a web in your husband's body. It tries to fasten it to as many parts of his body as possible. It's an invisible web. We can try and reduce the spider's activity, but the web remains. Do you understand? We call that a small-cell lung carcinoma. Not so long ago we couldn't do anything about it at all. In those days he would have been gone in two months. Now we have chemotherapy. That works in the sense that he is still here with us. He's alive. But we can't get rid of the cancer completely. It'll stay in his body. So it's pointless to keep doing scans to see if it's still there, because it's always there. But if he has complaints, then we do tests to see how we can reduce those complaints. What we are trying is to make the time that still remains as pleasant as possible for your husband.'

'Now I have my answer,' Mrs Dekker says quietly. 'Somehow I knew it, but they would never tell me directly.'

'I can understand that it is a difficult and uncertain time for you. I can't take away that uncertainty.' Ilona leans over the table and touches Mrs Dekker's shoulder. Mrs Dekker bows her head.

'With every little cough I worry. It was a terrible shock for us that it came back,' Mrs Dekker says.

'This kind of tumour never goes away,' Ilona repeats. 'It always reappears. In the case of your husband it's in his head. That's a typical pattern of development for this kind of tumour. What I mean is that your husband isn't the only one.'

The tears are streaming down Mrs Dekker's cheeks. 'I don't want to lose him,' she says. 'I want to keep him with me as long as possible. He's fighting but I'm so unsure.'

'Its difficult for you. It's difficult when you're sick, but it's sometimes worse when someone you love is sick.' Mrs Dekker nods.

'For me it's different,' Mr Dekker says. It is the first time he has spoken.

'Yes,' the doctor says. 'You're different. You have the illness and she doesn't. And women deal with these matters differently to men.'

Dr Racz examines Mr Dekker. Mr Dekker asks about the most recent X-rays. 'No change,' Dr Racz says.

'Then I think there must be an infection or something,' Mr Dekker says. 'I can feel something there.' Ilona Racz has another look at the X-rays. Then she puts the stethoscope to Mr Dekker's chest and listens.

'It's the tumour reappearing,' Mrs Dekker says.

'Don't be so negative, mum,' Mr Dekker says.

'I don't see anything on the X-ray,' Ilona says. 'But I can hear something at the spot where the tumour was. Something's not right there. It's a sensitive spot, and all kinds of things can happen there. We'll have to wait and see whether it's the tumour or not. It doesn't sound very reassuring, but we'll have to wait until something happens and then decide what to do about it.' The doctor's words have had a calming effect on Mr and Mrs Dekker. 'What do you do to keep yourself busy?' Ilona asks Mr Dekker.

'All kinds of things,' Mr Dekker answers. 'At the moment I'm in a rehabilitation centre because of my sugar. While I'm there I work on my hobby, upholstery.'

'And how are you otherwise? I gather you'd rather be at home than in the rehabilitation centre?'

'You have to understand, I'm someone who likes his freedom, always on the move, so sometimes . . .' his voice breaks.

'You just want to break out?'

'Exactly.' The atmosphere in the doctor's office is pleasant. Mrs Dekker has said what she wanted to say and, although it was hard, has heard what she needed to hear. The conversation switches to going home, children and birthdays. Mrs Dekker has another cry. Then Dr Racz brings the interview to an end. 'Okay, I suggest you come back again in six weeks. If there are complaints before that, then phone us. Who do you want to see next time, me or Dr Liem?'

'We don't mind,' Mrs Dekker says. 'At first I was unhappy that we couldn't see Liem, but this was a good discussion, so now I don't mind.' She wipes her eyes.

'We discuss everything anyway, so we both know the situation well,' the doctor assures her.

'I think you have to maintain trust in the doctor,' Mr Dekker says. 'Now we are also on good terms with the GP. It wasn't always like that. We've discussed things and settled our differences. He now calls in once a fortnight and spends half an hour with us.' Mr Dekker stands up. 'Let's make a move. We don't want to keep the doctor all day.'

A different attitude

Strolling back to the ward shortly before midday I hear footsteps behind me.

'Anne-Mei, Anne-Mei.' I turn round to see Ilona Racz.

'What did you think of the meeting with the Dekkers this morning?' she asks as she catches up with me.

'It was a good discussion,' I say. 'I think it was hard for them, but it was necessary. What was your impression?'

'Me too, me too. Everything got said that needed to be said. Mrs Dekker cried. At first it was because of anger and powerlessness, but later it was because of sadness.'

'Yes,' I say. 'It seemed as though she was relieved.'

'What I find difficult,' Ilona says, 'is the chemo and the hope that lingers. When I was training I often saw patients who had been admitted with a "dip" after chemotherapy, or a recurrence, patients with a very poor prognosis who spoke as though they still had a whole life before them. Amazing. I sometimes wondered what the doctors told them.' She shakes her head. 'If it were me I'd do things differently. I'd be much clearer about what was happening. I'd tell them that they were dying. But then I have a different attitude to Guido Liem.' She smiles. 'That's why I'd do things differently.'

'Is that the reason?' I ask.

'Definitely.'

'It's not often that a patient is told, "You're going to die".'

'No, not often.'

'I once heard Maarten Rutgers [one of the doctors] say to a patient who had asked what the choice was, "You're going to die or you're going to die," and then go on to talk about chemotherapy.'

'That's typical of Maarten,' Ilona says, smiling. 'Ach, I don't really have the wisdom either. I don't know what the best counselling method is. Maybe there are good reasons for letting people cherish hope. But I have the impression that giving hope also stems from doctors trying to protect themselves. Telling someone that they're going to die, giving up hope, flies in the face of the will to cure. Doctors like to pretend they have certainty. In fact, there's a lot we're uncertain about, but we don't like to admit it.'

The style of the doctor

In the first chapter I noted that doctors in the Ruysdael Clinic generally informed their patients in the same way. But I would be misrepresenting reality if I failed to devote some attention to individual variation. Ilona Racz is one of the doctors who is critical about the way oncology patients are informed about their illness. It was mainly the junior doctors like Ilona who had a problem when confronted with lung cancer patients who hoped for a cure. This made them wonder whether the patients had been properly counselled. One junior doctor told me she was pleased that she had now done part of her training on the lung cancer ward. Previously, in the Emergency Room, she had often been confronted with lung cancer patients who had a totally wrong picture of their prognosis and had found it difficult to understand where this came from. Junior doctors had the same experience of patients' hope as did the nurses and myself. It might have been coincidence, but among the junior doctors it was mainly the women who were critical about the way in which patients were counselled. Of the two research fellows with whom I worked it was also the woman who was critical of the way in which patients were informed.

Doctors have different individual styles of practice (see Pool 1998, 2000). One of the reasons for this is the differing ideas about what exactly their job entails. I have already noted that Drs Liem and Veerman did not consider the provision of psychosocial support for their patients as part of their job description. They saw their task as exclusively medical-technical. Doctor Racz, on the other hand, does consider this part of her job. I often saw her defending the interests of patients and their relatives. For example, she once arranged for a patient, who had gone into a coma during tests, to be sent to the chest ward where staff knew her rather than to the neurology ward specified in the rules. She had been present during that disastrous test and afterwards often spoke to the family about what had happened and how they were coping. The supervising specialist, on the other hand, never spoke to the family again (see The 1997a, Chapter 10).

But for Ilona Racz it is more than a simple question of job descriptions. She derives job satisfaction from the provision of psychosocial support to patients and their relatives. She is prepared to visit patients at home and she is willing to work after hours. I never saw Drs Liem and Veerman come back to the hospital in a weekend especially for a meeting with patients or relatives or to say goodbye to a patient. Both doctors were often in the hospital during the weekend, but that was in the service of science: to carry out laboratory research or write papers, both reasons that were unlikely to tempt Ilona Racz into the hospital during the weekend.

Marcel Heller was somewhere in between. He did not have the scientific ambitions of Ronald Veerman and Guido Liem and, unlike them, he did not have a PhD. But he was interested in research, and certainly more so than Ilona Racz. He visited patients on the ward more frequently than Drs Liem and Veerman; in fact, he visited the ward most afternoons to see how his patients were doing. This was highly valued by the nurses on the ward.

Patients also often asked the nurses why the outpatient clinic doctors were seen so infrequently on the wards and some felt the doctor had abandoned them. As a result of his visits, Marcel Heller had a good relationship with the ward nurses.

Sometimes it seemed as though Ilona Racz welcomed the role of psychosocial support provision. She was approachable for patients and was less formal and and less distanced than the specialists. She was more 'girlish'. Moreover, she seemed to hear the needs of patients and their relatives. She was immediately aware that Mrs Dekker was panicking and in need of time and attention. Mrs Dekker had phoned Dr Liem because she needed help, but Dr Liem had interpreted this as a routine consultation and let Ilona deal with it. Perhaps it is not so much a question of hearing need as *wanting* to hear. Ilona Racz was open to patients' problems and questions. But it goes further than that. Although Dr Liem was less proficient in dealing with patient's emotions than Ilona, he did notice when patients were having difficulties. Perhaps he sometimes chose to not see things. There are various reasons why he might do that: other priorities, shortage of time, not having a solution to the problem, clumsiness, self-protection.

This is a rather black-and-white presentation of things. Of course Dr Liem and Dr Veerman also gave psychosocial support to their patients. Later I describe how Mrs Wessels, whose husband was beyond treatment and dying in the care of the GP, regularly telephoned Dr Liem for advice. I have presented these differences to illustrate the way in which differences in doctors' interpretation of their role, different interests, characters and attitudes, all influence their styles of practice and the ways they inform patients.

Infection or progression?

[26 November] Dorien Meulman and I are talking when Marcel Heller enters the office carrying two X-rays. He hangs them up.

'What do you make of these?' he asks Dorien.

'Oh, progression.' She sighs. 'It's particularly clear in the lateral view.' She points to a patchy area.

Dr Heller nods. 'I agree.'

'Mr Wiersema?' Dr Meulman asks.

'Yes.'

'Good morning.' Guido Liem comes into the office.

'Guido, have a look at this?' Marcel invites.

Dr Liem sticks his hands in his pockets and bends over the X-rays.

'Yes, yes,' he says pensively. 'Progression? It could also be an infection. It's not entirely clear that it's progression. I'd give him antibiotics for a week and see what happens. Let him come back in a week, then it should be clear what's wrong. In the meantime we can do further tests.'

'Okay,' Marcel says as he puts away the X-rays.

'That'll also give him time to get used to the idea that something could be wrong,' Dr Liem continues. Everyone nods. 'And if it's progression then we can give him CDE.'

Marcel Heller picks up Mr Wiersema's file and turns to me, 'Let's go.' I follow him through the waiting room. On the way we pass Mr Wiersema. 'Are you coming?' Dr Heller asks him. He gets up and follows us.

'My wife will be with us shortly,' Mr Wiersema says. 'She's with Natasha,' he whispers to me. I nod but don't dare to look at him. I feel a traitor. How often has he entrusted me with his cares? I know how scared he is of the hospital. I know what he should know, but how can I tell him, with Dr Heller just in front of us? But if Dr Heller had not been there, would I have told him there, in the waiting room? He would have asked. Would I have remained silent? Or would I have simply avoided him?

Dr Heller hangs up the X-rays. Mr Wiersema follows his movements. 'I might as well tell you straight away,' Dr Heller says. 'The X-rays don't look good. Look, over here, it's become whiter.' Mr Wiersema looks disbelieving.

'I made this appointment myself,' he says. 'I haven't been feeling well the last couple of weeks. It's become worse the past few days. I can feel pressure in my chest.' Mr Wiersema is talking faster. 'At first I thought it was an infection,' he says hopefully, 'but the GP didn't give me any antibiotics.' He looks distraught.

'It's not entirely clear what's wrong,' Dr Heller says. There's something on the X-ray, but we're not sure what it is. We need to investigate. It might be an infection. That's why I want to try antibiotics. But it could also be something else. If it is an infection then the antibiotics should make you feel a lot better by next week. I also want to do some tests to see if we can find out what else it might be.'

'Is it the cancer?' Mr Wiersema asks.

'We don't know,' Dr Heller explains. 'That's what we have to find out.'

'But is it cancer?' Mr Wiersema asks again.

'We have to find that out,' the doctor repeats. 'But it is possible.'

Mr Wiersema looks shocked. 'Where is it exactly?' he wants to know. 'It's cancer, isn't it?' he asks, looking at me. 'My wife is always here with me, but she's not here,' he says. 'I have to go and find her.' He gets up, perspiration forming on his forehead.

'Let me go,' I say, and I go into the waiting room. I see Mrs Wiersema and she waves when she sees me. I do not know what I must say, what I can say, what I am allowed to say. 'We're inside talking,' I say, not answering her smile. 'Are you going to join us?' She follows me back to the surgery, looking worried.

'It's not good,' Mr Wiersema says immediately as we enter. She covers her mouth with her hand. Dr Heller explains.

'If it is a tumour, then it'll be finished before Christmas, won't it?' Mr Wiersema asks.

'If there's something there then we definitely need to make a plan about what to do,' Dr Heller says.

After the meeting I go and sit in a corner of the waiting room with Mr and Mrs Wiersema. I am in the middle. They both start talking to me simultaneously. Is it an infection? What was it that the doctor said exactly? Can it be a tumour? What do I think? Mr Wiersema gets up and disappears into the toilet with the paper cup Dr Heller has given him for a sputum sample. When he has gone we see Mr Dekker at the other end of the waiting room. He raises his hand in greeting and we wave back.

'Joop is having a hard time facing Dekker,' Mrs Wiersema says quietly. 'I like to call them, but I do it when he's not around. It's too confrontational otherwise. I don't want to believe that things are going wrong. He does. He's scared. He went to see Natasha yesterday and she said quite explicitly that he didn't have metastases.' She looks at me triumphantly. I nod. 'He still does everything,' she continues. 'He jogs, he paints.' She shakes her head. 'It's just not possible.'

Mr Wiersema returns. 'I've so many questions,' he says. 'I need information, I need to talk.' He stares at the floor. 'You know,' he says to me. 'I wish I could just phone Heller at home one evening and talk. We've just seen him, I know, but I already have all kinds of other things I want to ask him.'

Mr Koster's daughter arrives with Mr and Mrs Bokjes. I feel Mr and Mrs Wiersema hoping that they will not stop and ask how he is. Sandra Koster stops and shakes hands. 'Things are not going well with Dekker,' she says. Mr and Mrs Wiersema nod silently. Mr Bokjes is jolly and talkative. He and his wife are always happy to see people they know in the waiting room. Mr Bokjes has recovered and his face is no longer swollen and red.

St Nicholas

[5 December] It is drizzling as I cycle through the hospital grounds on my way home. I see a man on a bicycle waving at me. I cycle over and see it is Mr Wiersema. 'I've just had a scan,' he shouts as I approach. As we stand at the roadside, astride our bicycles he tells me about all the tests he has undergone in the past week.

'It's been a good thing,' he says. 'It means I didn't have time to worry. In the weekend I was at home and I was agitated. They think there's a blood clot somewhere in my brain and that that's the cause of my numbness.'

'Oh,' I say. 'Are you still decorating?'

'Yes, I've almost finished. Listen,' he says more quietly, bending toward me. 'I'm doing it for my wife and the children. Then at least that's been done.' He avoids eye contact. 'Because you never know.'

It has started to rain more heavily. There is the sound of music, and a *Sinterklaas* procession comes down the road. *Sinterklaas*, St Nicholas, is the Dutch equivalent of Father Christmas. He appears at the beginning of December, dressed in red bishop's robes and accompanied by a group of helpers, made up in black minstrel style, called *Zwarte Pieten*, 'Black Peters'. One of the *Pieten* has a large ghetto blaster on his shoulder, from which issues shrill *Sinterklaas* music.

'Hello *Sinterklaas*,' Mr Wiersema calls.

'Good afternoon sir,' *Sinterklaas* answers solemnly.

'This is Anne-Mei,' Mr Wiersema tells *Sinterklaas*. 'Come over here,' he says to me, pulling my sleeve. He leans forward and whispers into the saintly ear.

'So,' *Sinterklaas* says to me. 'I hear that you are always so friendly to the patients in the hospital.' He turns to one of his helpers. '*Piet*, give this girl some *pepernoten*.' I receive my handful of the small, traditional, ginger flavoured biscuits, and the procession moves on.

'I'll be off as well,' Mr Wiersema says. 'Have to get back to the missus and tell her of the day's events. Are you going to be at the clinic tomorrow?' he asks. I say I will. 'See you then,' he says, and cycles away.

'Give my regards to your wife,' I shout over my shoulder, and he sticks his arm in the air. It is still raining.

Metastases in the brain

[2 December] The next morning I sit next to Dr Liem, opposite Mr and Mrs Wiersema. They are both silent and tense.

'I don't have any results yet,' Dr Liem says, looking through the papers in front of him. 'The X-rays don't give a very clear picture. There's something white and that's . . . that's the beginning of . . . what?' He looks at the X-rays again. 'The white patch hasn't become any bigger since last week.'

'What about the scan?' Mr Wiersema asks.

'Let me phone,' Dr Liem says. He picks up the phone and dials. 'Guido Liem here. I have a Mr Wiersema here with me, number 7734. Yesterday a scan was made of his head. Is there any result?' He listens for a few minutes. 'Mmm, yes, thank you.' He hangs up and looks gravely at the couple opposite him. 'On the scan there is a tumour visible in the brain,' he says. An unpleasant silence descends on the room. Mr Wiersema turns pale and begins to perspire. 'I'm feeling warm,' he says. Mrs Wiersema begins to cry. 'You try and control yourself as long as possible,' she says apologetically to the doctor. I get her a cup of water and hand her a tissue. She looks at me through the tears, a mixture of helplessness and gratitude. 'You're so nice,' she says.

'I realize this is difficult for you,' Dr Liem says. 'It's unpleasant news. I think we need to discuss further on Monday. I need to see all the other test results first. But you can assume that what I have just told you is correct. When we have the other results we need to discuss chemotherapy. You have to think about it over the weekend and decide whether you want to continue with treatment.'

'Have I got a chance?' Mr Wiersema asks, his fists clenched on the table.

'Certainly,' Dr Liem answers. 'Otherwise I wouldn't suggest it in the first place. Take your time and think it over. We'll discuss it on Monday.'

'We don't need to think about it,' Mr Wiersema says immediately. We'll persevere. I'll fight on to the bitter end.'

'He's no good at waiting,' Mrs Wiersema says. 'He gets agitated. Last week-end was terrible. Waiting drives him mad.'

'Well,' Dr Liem says, taking some forms from a drawer. 'If you're sure, then I can apply for the treatment immediately.' Mr and Mrs Wiersema nod vigorously.

'So you do give me a chance?' Mr Wiersema asks again.

'Certainly.'

'Our son is going overseas,' Mrs Wiersema says. 'Is that okay?'

'Yes, that's fine,' Dr Liem says.

'So I've got at least four weeks?' Mr Wiersema asks hopefully.

'I can't guarantee anything,' the doctor replies. 'Listen,' he says, laying down his fountain pen. 'Funny things can happen. Even with me. I can walk out of the hospital this afternoon straight under a bus.' Mr and Mrs Wiersema nod. 'You have an aggressive tumour,' he continues. You've been coming here since February. If we hadn't done anything you wouldn't be here now. I would have given you three months at most.'

'So if I hadn't had the chemotherapy then I wouldn't be here?'

'Right. And the same thing applies again now. There are doctors who prefer to do nothing in situations like this, but I personally think that's unacceptable. I would like to continue.' He proceeds to fill in the forms.

'I'm a wreck,' Mr Wiersema says. I've never been so bad.' He asks again about his chances.

'This type of tumour reacts well to chemotherapy,' Dr Liem says. 'After two courses we'll check to see if it's working. If it isn't then we'll stop. And even in that case there are still other things we can do. But I have to tell you, the possibilities are becoming more limited.'

The realization of truth

Following on from the second bad news interview with Mr Wiersema I want to return to the doctors' pattern of information provision. In the case of Mr Dekker I remarked on the gradual nature of the process. Mr Wiersema's case illustrates that this is not simply a consequence of practical considerations. The doctors must await the test results before they can say anything with certainty. But they also use this consciously as a counselling strategy. Dr Liem advises Dr Heller to mention the possibility of a recurrence so that Mr Wiersema can get used to the idea.

The provision of information follows a specific course of development. In the first consultation the doctor prepares the patient for probable bad news ('it *could* be a recurrence') and arranges for tests. The possibility of further therapy is also often mentioned ('Then you can decide what you want to do'). During the next meeting the doctor's suspicions are confirmed by the test results and therapy is offered.

Just as in the first bad news interview, doctors do not discuss details of the prognosis. Doctors do mention that the recurrence has made the patient's chances worse, however. Unlike in the first bad news interview, Mr Wiersema, like most patients, does actively try to find out how much time he has left. He tries to force Dr Heller to give a time by making suggestions himself ('It'll be finished before Christmas, won't it?'). The answers he gets are general. Initially Dr Heller tries to avoid answering and focus attention on the therapy. When Mr Wiersema insists, this time with Dr Liem, the doctor reflects on the illness process and gives a global overview of the situation. No precise prognosis is given. The doctor neutralizes the prognosis by comparing the patient's situation with his own: he could also die suddenly (see Costain Schou 1993; de Swaan 1985).

The first explanation that doctors give for this is that it is difficult to make accurate predictions because so many factors are involved. There are patients who survive much longer than doctors could have hoped (Mr Wessels, for example) and there are patients who die unexpectedly. But these are exceptional, and doctors could say something about prognosis if they wanted to. How long a patient still had left was a common subject of discussion between doctors and nurses, for example.

The second reason that doctors give for their reluctance to discuss prognosis with patients is that a precise death sentence would have a numbing effect on them and that they would then focus on a date and spend their time counting the days (see Wagener 1996).

Dr Heller and Dr Racz put an end to the fearful speculations and uncertainty of Mr Wiersema and Mrs Dekker. The truth is told, the hope of cure dashed and the fearful suspicions confirmed. I focus on Mr Wiersema and Mrs Dekker because in this phase of the illness they are receptive to the doctor's terrible news. Earlier in the process doctors describe the course of the illness and label it incurable. The difference is not so much that the doctors tell more of the truth in a later phase but rather that patients and their relatives understand more.

The doctor tells Mr Wiersema that his most recent complaints are the result of a recurrence. Up until then he had tried to distance himself from what was happening to Mr Dekker. He now comes to realize that he is just as vulnerable and that what is happening to Mr Dekker is what also awaits himself. His experience of physical decline, the example of Mr Dekker and the doctors' words all coincide in this phase.

Dr Racz tells Mrs Dekker that her husband will not get better. Other doctors had told her this previously: Dr Kooiman during the first bad news interview and Dr Liem in the second. But it was only when Dr Racz talked to her that she seemed to realize fully what she was being told. An important factor here is that the message was repeated. Dr Racz used a different terminology, one that was closer to the experiences of Mrs Dekker, and she took the time to sit and discuss the matter with her. In this meeting Dr Racz put an end to the discrepancy between what Mrs Dekker saw and what she heard.

The confrontational meeting with Mr Dekker

[8 December] Mr Wiersema is receiving the final infusion in his course of chemotherapy. When he is called into the infusion room, Mrs Wiersema stays in the waiting room with me. The news that the cancer had returned had been a huge blow. They had been prepared for news that his lungs were bad, but not for a tumour in the brain.

'Joop's been to see Natasha,' Mrs Wiersema says. 'But she talked her way out of it. She said that she had felt something, but hadn't really taken much notice because she was concentrating on his lungs and not on his head.'

'So it took you completely by surprise?' I ask. She nods.

'What happened to Dekker did make us think, of course. Klaas Dekker phoned on Saturday and Joop answered the phone himself. Dekker doesn't talk about himself, he always says "we". *We're* turning over the final page of our lives; *we're* living from day to day. When Klaas talks like that then Joop gets really upset. We've agreed that he won't answer the phone any more. He can't cope with calls like that. On Wednesday we discussed Dekker with Dr Liem. He said that Dekker was a completely different case. That calmed Joop down. If the doctor says so . . . understand?

'Dekker and his wife rarely talk about death. They're in that phase. They've shed their tears and now want to enjoy as much as possible. So that she and the children can retain a good feeling about this time. Then at least they have the jokes and the good times to remember.

'Joop is strong, as long as he avoids other patients. He talks to the children and he's positive. We know that the options are now limited. I see things differently to in the beginning. We hope that this treatment works and that it will extend the time he has left, but we no longer talk about getting better. We stopped that when we saw all the others deteriorating, one by one. When Dekker heard he had a brain tumour we said to each other, "That's not a good sign".

'Waiting is the worst for Joop. Dr Liem interpreted the situation correctly last week when he applied for the treatment immediately. Joop only really calmed down when he was receiving the infusion. At least then something's being done.'

Reunion in the waiting room

[17 December, 8:15 am] I hurry through the waiting room when I hear someone calling me. I turn to see Mr and Mrs Wiersema waving. They are over in a corner, away from their usual place among the other patients. Mr Wiersema calls for me to come and join them, and as I approach he moves up so that I can take my usual seat between them. Things are not going well. Mr Wiersema says he now knows what it means to be short of breath. 'Mrs Dekker phoned,' Mr Wiersema tells me. 'Dekker's having a hard time. They're bringing him in for a check-up today, on a trolley. He can't walk.'

Mr Wiersema has to go for X-rays. Mrs Wiersema stays with me in the waiting room. She tells me about the discussion with Mrs Dekker. 'Rietje has accepted that he's going to die,' she says. 'They know he's not going to get better. Klaas had asked Rietje to phone to see how we were. He'd seen Joop in the waiting room and suspected that things weren't good. That was the day Joop heard that things weren't good and that Joop saw us but didn't join us, remember? He wanted to apologize. I didn't want to tell Joop at first, but when I heard that Dekker was being brought in on a trolley I had to tell him. Otherwise it might have been a shock. Joop's starting to doubt Natasha. I didn't believe in her at all in the beginning. But she did anticipate things that later happened. I thought it was good for Joop, for his peace of mind. But there was a problem. Natasha said that Joop shouldn't accept radiotherapy. Now the doctors have said that he needs radiotherapy. He wanted me to tell Natasha, but I told him it was better if he told her himself. Natasha didn't mind, because it was only a small tumour. Joop's loosing his trust in her and he now relies more on the hospital.'

I suggest a cup of coffee and walk over to the coffee machine at the other end of the waiting room. While I am waiting for the plastic cups to fill I feel a hand on my arm. I turn to see Mr Koster, sporting a head of new hair. Over his shoulder I see Mr Fresco shuffle into the waiting room on the arm of his fiancée. From the reception desk a beaming Mr and Mrs Bokjes wave. To the left Mr and Mrs Heuvel are in conversation with Mrs Fisher-Rijn. And Mr Dekker is expected at any moment. It seems like a waiting room reunion. Then I see Mr Wiersema, X-rays in hand, shuffle nervously into the waiting room. He makes a detour around the other patients and rejoins his wife. It is a reunion to which Mr Wiersema is not invited.

An hour later Dr Heller sees Mr Wiersema. He carries out an extensive physical examination. Mr Wiersema says he feels terrible. He can no longer manage the decorating work at home. He feels weaker and weaker. Walking has become difficult. Dr Heller thinks he might have bronchitis and that this is part of the problem. 'All those pills,' Mr Wiersema sighs. 'I'm sick of all the pills.' At the end of the consultation Mr and Mrs Wiersema wish us a merry Christmas. As they close the door behind them, Dr Heller sighs, 'and a merry Christmas to you too.' He looks at me and raises his eyebrows. 'It'll be their last,' he says.

The confrontation with other patients and defence mechanisms

Here I would like to dwell on a phenomenon that has already been mentioned: rehearsal. After Mr Dekker was diagnosed with brain metastases he and his wife maintained telephone contact with the Wiersemas. Mr Wiersema found this very confrontational. He couldn't sleep the night after Mr Dekker had said that *they* were turning over the final page of their lives. They agree not to answer the phone, but in the hospital waiting room it was more difficult to avoid fellow sufferers. 'Initially we enjoyed contact with the others,' Mrs Wiersema told me. 'But now we can't stand listening to their stories. We have our hands full coping with our own problems.' Avoidance is a defence mechanism. Another defence mechanism is 'downward social comparison,' in which patients are able to evaluate their situation positively by comparing themselves with others who are apparently worse off (Costain Schou 1993). Mr Wiersema and Mr Koster continually tried to reduce their own anxiety by comparing themselves to Mr Dekker. 'Klaas has metastases in his neck, but I've only got them in my liver,' Mr Koster said.

Mr and Mrs Wiersema said that if they were able to do things over again they would not have established such intensive contacts with other patients. Here it is necessary to place this in a wider context. When their illnesses are in the same phase then patients feel comfortable supporting each other, but when one's illness develops faster then contact is confrontational for the one who is 'lagging behind'. If he later catches up, then contact is once more a possibility. And after they have died, their widows can understand and support each other. Most patients and their partners agreed that contact with others could be confrontational, but were generally positive about their contact with others when they reflected on the illness trajectory as a whole (Buunk et al. 1990).

Mr Koster's recurrence

Mr Koster tells Dr Heller that he does not feel his old self yet. He almost loses his balance a few times as he gets undressed for his physical examination. Otherwise he is okay, he says. He is not afraid to come to the hospital. 'I consider this a routine check-up,' he says, almost indifferently. Because I spent so much time with Mrs Wiersema in the waiting room I have missed the preparatory discussion with Dr Heller. I listen and at the same time try to read Dr Heller's notes. I am shocked to see 'local recurrence' written under the heading 'conclusion'.

'Mr Koster,' Dr Heller says as he moves over to the X-rays. 'I want us to have a look at these X-rays together, because I'm not happy with them at all.' He explains that the tumour has reappeared in exactly the same place. The news comes as a bolt out of the blue. Mr Koster and his daughter Sandra stare at the floor and say nothing. 'We have to act quickly,' Dr Heller resumes after a while. 'I suggest that we start today.'

'No no,' Mr Koster waves away the doctor's suggestion. 'Monday is a much better day. I see this as a preparatory discussion, and Monday is early enough.' He looks at me. 'This is not very nice news,' he says.

'Dr Heller,' Sandra says. 'What will it be like after this new treatment? Will dad's cancer ever be completely cured?'

Dr Heller shakes his head. 'Now that the tumour has come back, his prospects have worsened,' he says.

Back in the waiting room Mr Koster keeps repeating, 'Once you've got cancer you never get rid of it.' He looks straight in front of him and leans on his walking stick. Sandra sits next to him and stares. Tears stream down her cheeks. Mr Koster stares at the taxi driver who has come to pick him up. 'See you on Monday,' he says, without looking at me.

The fear of emotions

After the outpatient clinic I join the nurses for lunch in the canteen. I talk about all I have experienced. Carola Vroom, one of the nurses, listens attentively to my story. 'It's such a pity,' she says, 'that doctors always find it necessary to resort to chemotherapy. Sometimes they aren't even sure it extends the patient's life. I spoke to a patient and his wife the other day. They told me that it was really difficult to choose every time they were offered therapy. They had the feeling that they had to accept, otherwise they had the niggling doubt that maybe they hadn't done everything possible. They knew that he wouldn't get better, but each course of therapy meant that he could spend a few more weeks with his family. I wish the doctors didn't confront people with that choice. I wish they said, "Sorry, just go home and make the best of the situation, and we'll help you with that." But no, they have to offer something every time. And it's difficult to refuse. Sometimes they accept for the relatives, so they can be together a bit longer. They almost always accept.'

'Why do you think they accept?'

'It's the hospital, isn't it? Maybe because it's an academic hospital, doctors feel the need to treat. It worries me more and more. What are we doing, for God's sake?'

'So why do you think doctors are so obsessed with treatment?' I ask.

'Their training. Treatment and scientific research are their priorities. Maybe they're also scared to discuss the issue, scared to tell the patient, scared of the patient's emotions. It's difficult to cope with the feeling of being powerless. I have difficulty with it myself. When a patient says to me, "I have to agree to chemo-therapy, otherwise I'll die," I would also find it difficult to answer, "You're going to die anyway." So I think the doctors' fear is an important factor.'

The magical power of treatment

Patients and their relatives trust the power or medical technology. Medical science develops rapidly. The outpatient clinic waiting room reverberated with talk of all kinds of wonders. Understandable, because had the doctors not said that a mere ten years ago there had not even been any treatment for the small-cell lung carcinoma? And look how far we have come in those ten years. Many silently hoped that they would be one of the select few who were cured. But you never knew, perhaps the doctors had another, even more powerful therapy that they were waiting to deploy at the right moment. Or maybe some new wonder cure would be discovered just in time.

For many patients and their relatives treatment was much more than a medical-technical affair. I have already described how important it was for patients that 'something' was happening. Sometimes I had the impression that it did not make much difference what the treatment was, as long as 'something' was being done.

Nothing is worse for patients than waiting passively. I often encountered patients, like Mr Wiersema, who, quite literally, only became calm when they were on the receiving end of a chemotherapy infusion. Therapy, or rather the idea that something was being done, had a pacifying, almost magical effect on the patient's mood. Treatment made emotions controllable.

I have already mentioned that nothing can cheer a patient up more than a doctor saying that he has nothing to worry about, or that he is satisfied with the result of treatment. What the doctor says is more important than what the patient feels. Responsibility for the patient and the illness lies with the doctor, and the mere presence of a doctor can make the patient feel better. In Chapter 2 Dr Liem referred to this as the doctor's aura.

Nuland gives a wonderful description of the feeling of security that he experienced as a child in the mere presence of the GP. It was not so much medical knowledge as the magical aura that made him dream of becoming a doctor.

Before there were two digits in my age, I had seen the hope (I choose the word deliberately) that a doctor's presence brings to a worried family. There were several frightening emergencies during my mother's long illness, even in the years before she had begun her descent to death. The mere knowledge that someone had gone to the drugstone phone to call the doctor, and the word that he was on the way, changed the atmosphere in our small apartment from terrified helplessness to a secure sense that someone who stepped across the threshold with a smile and an air of competence, who called each of us by name, who understood that beyond anything else we needed reassurance, and whose

very entrance into our home conveyed it – that was the man I wanted
to be.

(Nuland 1995: 247)

At the beginning of the twentieth century the young Nuland placed the
family doctor on a pedestal. The adult cancer patients in my study did the
same with their specialist at the end of the century.

Patients have an interest in looking up to the doctor. It is easy to believe
someone who is prestigious. The more prestige, the more credibility.
Van Dantzig compares the older medical profession with the modern
specializations that deal with patients with a poor prognosis. A hundred
years ago, when medicine was still relatively ineffective, the social prestige
of the profession was high. This was based not on the actual efficacy but on
the pretension of efficacy. The doctor dealt in hope and in order to sell
hope the consumer – the patient – had to believe. And in order to believe
there had to be authority (van Dantzig 1993). The specialists in this study
cannot offer their patients cure. The most they can offer is an extension of
life by one or two years at most. This is a lot more than in the past, but still
less than what patient's want: cure.

We pin our hopes on the doctor because of a deeply rooted resistance to
mortality and a related inability to cope with dying. Doctors give patients
hope, sometimes without realizing it, sometimes against their own better
judgement (de Swaan 1985; Ter Borg 1993). The mere offer of therapy gives
the patient hope. Patients feel the need to try everything that is offered. The
thought that they might not have tried all the options is unbearable. Tijmstra
(1987) refers to this as anticipated decision regret.

A study was carried out in another hospital to explore why patients agree
to participate in a phase 1 trial that doctors explicitly said would have no
therapeutic effect. In spite of this patients agreed to participate in the hope
of some individual therapeutic effect. The need to 'do something' also played
a role (Brinkman-Woltjer et al. 1988). In this way medical action contains
patients' fear of death and obliges their drive to live (Elias 1990).

9 No therapy for Mr Wessels

Mr Wessels has a recurrence

[4 October] 'The developments in the case of Mr Wessels are not satisfactory,' Dr Liem is saying. 'He is still having the attacks, and the question is whether they are a result of the brain metastases or the medication.' He looks at the X-rays and sighs. 'Recurrence.' He reads in Mr Wessels's file. 'Diagnosed a year ago with a small-cell lung carcinoma. Brain metastases. Received CDE chemotherapy. Recurrence three months after the last course of treatment. Has shaking limbs. Occasionally loses consciousness and can't remember the attacks afterwards. Receiving second-line chemotherapy. Had fourth course of carboplatin on the 13th of September, and so there is now progression.' He looks up from the file. 'Let's call him in,' he says.

Mr Wessels enters the room eating a sandwich. He greets us with a roguish smile, his mouth full of bread.

'Jan, please,' his wife admonishes, while trying to conceal a smile.

'We had to wait so long I got hungry,' he explains as he takes another bite.

Dr Liem is serious. He smiled about the sandwich, but he wants a change of mood. 'Why don't you put your sandwich down for a moment so that we can talk?' he suggests. When Mr Wessels has complied he asks, 'So how are you?'

'I'm okay,' Mr Wessels answers. 'I haven't had any more attacks.'

'If you take off your shirt I'll have a listen,' Dr Liem says. While he is undressing Dr Liem asks Mrs Wessels how she thinks he is doing.

'I don't know,' she says, hesitant. 'He's . . . err . . .' She points an index finger to her temple. 'Understand?' Dr Liem nods. 'He does strange things. Phones all kinds of people to ask things. He phoned a barber and asked him to come to the house to cut his hair. And the man came as well. On Saturday there was a party. We had to be smart. He bought a bow tie in a shop in the village. When he put it on he couldn't get it right, so he phoned the shop and had them come to the house and do it for him.' Dr Liem nods understandingly. Mr Wessels shrugs. 'It's the normal thing to do, isn't it?'

'And all those people come as well,' Mrs Wessels says admiringly. 'He gets them to come.'

'Yes, with a bit of charm you can achieve a lot,' Dr Liem says.

'Sometimes he's obsessed with time,' Mrs Wessels continues. 'I don't understand. He complains that time is moving too quickly. I change the clocks to calm him down. But it doesn't help.'

Dr Liem takes Mr Wessels's pulse. 'One side is faster than the other,' Mr Wessels says.

'That's normal' says Dr Liem. He hangs his stethoscope round his neck, washes his hands and takes his place behind his desk. 'I'll get straight to the point,' he says. 'The tumour has grown, in spite of the chemotherapy.' Mr Wessels is buttoning his shirt. The colour drains from Mrs Wessels's face, but she sits quietly opposite the doctor. This contrasts with her behaviour at the first diagnosis, when she shouted and blamed everyone.

'We can do two things,' Dr Liem says. 'We can wait and see or we can try another course of treatment. It depends on you, whether you want to try more treatment. What do you think?'

'I was glad that the treatment was finished,' Mr Wessels sighs. 'I've had enough of chemotherapy.'

'I can imagine,' Dr Liem says.

'The last time we were here things were still okay,' Mrs Wessels says. 'Things change so quickly.'

'Yes, that's the bad thing about this kind of cancer,' says Dr Liem. 'It grows very quickly.'

'If we don't do anything, will it keep growing?' Mrs Wessels asks.

'Yes it will.'

'And then . . . ?'

'Then there's not much time. A couple of months.'

'Then we have to do it,' she says resolutely. 'Jan, come and sit down and listen.'

'I've had enough of treatment,' Mr Wessels says. 'I was so glad it was finished, I don't like it,' he whines.

'Yes, but if we don't do anything then the tumour will continue to grow,' his wife explains.

'You have to decide yourself,' Dr Liem says. 'But I suggest that if you do decide to go for therapy then we must start today.'

'Can't we start next week?' Mr Wessels asks.

'What for?' his wife asks. 'If we have to do it then better to do it now. Why wait?'

'If you decide to take the treatment then we'll give you two courses and then decide whether to continue or not,' Dr Liem says. 'That will depend on how the tumour reacts to therapy. We'll check that on the X-rays.' He looks questioningly at the couple.

'Come on, Jan,' Mrs Wessels says. 'We'll go and have a bite to eat and then come back for the therapy.'
'If I have to then I suppose I have to,' whines Mr Wessels.

Preparing patients for brain metastases

Mr Wessels's recurrence is a variation on the well-known theme of brain metastases. Brain metastases are accompanied by a whole range of symptoms. The symptoms that 'my' patients experienced included loss of the ability to walk or talk, numbness on one side of the body, a superior vena cava syndrome, attacks of epilepsy, becoming dazed and disoriented. Mr Wessels adds to this list personality change. These are all unexpected, frightening and humiliating symptoms. It makes me wonder whether small-cell lung carcinoma patients should not be warned of the possibility of brain metastases beforehand. After all, the disease is known for its propensity to metastasize in the brain. Indeed, most of the patients in my study developed metastases there. As we have seen in the case of Mr Dekker and Mr Bokjes, this can be an incomprehensible and frightening experience. Because they often did not associate the symptoms with lung cancer, patients often did not act immediately. They struggled on by themselves and then went, like Mr Bokjes, to the GP rather than to the hospital.

Preparing patients for the manner in which the disease can develop would lead to earlier treatment, which is what doctors insist is so important. But a more important reason is that it would save patients and their partners a lot of suffering. I sometimes had the impression that if patients had known about the possibility of brain metastases it would have given them more of a feeling of control over the situation. When I mentioned this to doctors they rejected it. If they warned patients about the possibility of metastases in the brain then they would also have to inform them about the possibility of metastases in other organs. Small-cell lung carcinoma also frequently spreads to the liver and the bones. Telling patients about all possibilities would make them worry unnecessarily, doctors said. They would interpret every little ache and pain as a sign of the cancer spreading. They did not convince me that it was not a good idea to inform patients about the possibility of brain metastases, as their symptoms are more frightening and humiliating that those of metastases elsewhere.

'Now I understand what the doctor meant'

[3 November] Mr Wessels lies on a trolley in a hospital room. He looks in bad shape. His face is swollen. Mrs Wessels stands next to him. I ask how he feels and he shakes his head. 'Not very well,' he says. 'I'm deteriorating.'

'He's had a course of treatment,' his wife tells me. Last week we were keen to see whether there was any difference on the X-rays, whether the treatment was working. Because that would determine whether or not we continued. Dr Liem wasn't there so we saw Dr Heller. He didn't tell us what he saw on the X-rays. He said that Jan needed a blood transfusion, though. I asked him what the position was regarding the next course of treatment, but he couldn't tell us anything. "We'll have to see next week," he said. Then we had to wait in the corridor for hours because there weren't any beds available. Finally Jan ended up in the women's clinic. Dr Heller promised to come and see us, but he hasn't. We've been very upset. Dr Heller doesn't look you in the eye when he talks to you, and I don't like that. We have so many worries at the moment; we need attention. I phoned Dr Liem and asked whether we can see him in future. He said it was okay. I don't care if we have to wait three hours; I'd rather have Dr Liem. The therapy has made him sicker. He doesn't want any more. He'd rather live another two months as he is than six months with chemotherapy. At least now he can watch football on TV and talk to me.'

'I'll take every day that's given to me, that's how I see it,' Mr Wessels says.

'These days we talk a lot together, in a way we've never done before,' she says. 'He's so sweet.' She looks at her husband and then at me. 'I've accepted that this is it. When Dr Liem said the choice was between chemotherapy or two months I suddenly realized how serious the situation was.'

'Didn't you realize before that?' I ask.

'How should I put it? I knew and at the same time I didn't know. The doctor had already said that Jan had a brain tumour and wouldn't get better. Then they started talking about treatment. I thought, thank God, they can do something, and I held on to that. Later on I thought, he'll get better, otherwise they wouldn't go to all that trouble. His condition improved and things went well. I had hope. I thought, things are going to be okay. But on the day that Dr Liem said that the tumour was back I realized what the situation really was.'

'I realized earlier, when I was on the ward, but she didn't want to accept it,' Mr Wessels says.

'I might sound strange,' she says. 'But now we talk quite openly about death. We discuss things like whether burial or cremation is better. We're trying to arrange things as much as possible.'

Mr Wessels is becoming agitated. 'How many of you work here anyway?' he asks.

'It's his birthday next week,' Mrs Wessels says. 'The thirteenth. He wants to treat everyone, the girls from the infusion room, those from reception, Dr Liem and you. That's all, no one else. The children and grandchildren will also be there. We're hoping it'll be a nice day. I've ordered Indonesian food; he likes Indonesian food. I hope he'll still be able to eat it.

'A lot has changed between us during the last few months,' she resumes. He was always the strong man who did everything. He organized everything for me, financially as well. Now I have to take over and he has difficulty with that. Sometimes he tries to keep me under his thumb. That's when the bomb bursts.'

Mr Wessels wants to stop treatment

The door opens and Dr Liem enters with a file under his arm. 'How are things?' he asks.

'Not very good,' says Mr Wessels, sitting up with difficulty. He shows Dr Liem some painful patches on his arms and legs. Dr Liem is considerate. He examines the patches and fiddles a bit. Mrs Wessels complains that she cannot understand why they discharged her husband after his blood transfusion.

'I heard you had to wait in the corridor for a long time,' Dr Liem says. 'I'm sorry.'

'And then we were sent home, with antibiotics for the white blood cells,' she continues.

'No,' Dr Liem says. 'We prescribed the antibiotics for an infection. The white blood cells haven't recovered fully yet. Which means that we can't give him the second course of treatment yet so . . .'

Both Mr and Mrs Wessels try to interrupt him, but Dr Liem continues, 'So we'll have to postpone it for a week. But there is also the question of whether we should continue with the therapy,' he says, anticipating their interjection. Mrs Wessels raises her arms in the air. 'Just look at him,' she says. 'What are we doing?'

'It's just making me sicker,' Mr Wessels says. 'I don't want any more.'

'He says he'd rather have only two months as he is than longer with chemotherapy,' Mrs Wessels adds.

'Okay, that's clear,' Dr Liem says nodding. 'This is what we'll do. You come back in a week. We'll make another X-ray and check your blood. Then we can discuss further. In the meantime you can rest and think things over. If you still feel you want to stop treatment then we'll give it up. If you feel worse next week and it's difficult to come in to the hospital, then call me and we'll discuss over the phone.' Dr Liem offers his hand, thus closing the interview. Mrs Wessels pulls his sleeve.

'There's something I want to ask you,' she whispers. 'I want to know what will happen next.'

'I understand,' Dr Liem says. 'I can see that your husband is deteriorating rapidly.'

'I want to know what's going to happen,' she repeats. 'It's always such a shock when something happens. I want to know what it is and what I have to do. Can you tell me?'

'I think your husband will continue to deteriorate rapidly,' Dr Liem says. 'You have to be prepared for that. He might have another attack. Don't be afraid, just let it run its course. But it can happen rapidly.'

'I assume we can spend Christmas together,' she says hopefully. 'The children are coming.'

Dr Liem looks doubtful. 'Christmas is a long way off,' he says. I wouldn't count on it too much, although I can't tell you for certain.'

'It's almost his birthday. We want to make it a nice day.' The doctor nods. 'Do you think he'll have much pain? Will he suffer?'

'I don't think so.'

'Will he be gone suddenly?'

'I think he will.'

'I've accepted what's to come. We're having a good time together, we discuss everything, and we talk about death.'

'Good. And if there are things you need to organize then you should do that now.'

'Yes,' Mrs Wessels nods.

'Good luck,' Dr Liem says and walks away. Mrs Wessels turns to me.

'Of course, I want to keep him with me as long as possible. When the doctor told me what the situation really was, I wanted him to have the therapy. But what with the way he is, I can't force him. It would be selfish. It has to be his decision.'

The patient as expert

An obvious difference between the choice for first- and second-line chemotherapy is that some patients openly express doubts about the usefulness of the latter. By the time they have to make a decision about second-line therapy they have already experienced the side effects and the disappointment that they have not been cured. In other words, the experience of first-line therapy has turned the patients into 'experts'. They know what treatment entails and can make a more informed choice.

When Mr Wessels expressed doubt about second-line therapy after Dr Liem had informed him of the recurrence, this was not unusual. The way in which he allowed himself to be persuaded to accept treatment by Dr Liem and his wife was also not unusual. Patients are almost always influenced by their family in their decision to accept therapy.[1]

Patients who are adamant about refusing treatment risk falling into a 'medical snare'.[2] Doctors say convincingly that therapy produces good

---

1 See for example The (1997a, Chapter 3) in which a patient confides to a nurse that she has agreed to treatment because her husband and children wanted her to. After the discussion with the nurse and subsequent discussions with her family she finally decided to refuse treatment.

2 The term and its explanation are taken from a presentation by Dunning at a congress of the Psycho-geriatric Union in Utrecht, February 1998.

results. They then mention that the patient can try one or two courses of therapy without obligation before deciding whether or not to continue. At the same time the relatives pressurize the patient to try the therapy. The patient thinks, 'Why not? I've got nothing to lose; maybe it will help'. And in any case, refusal raises the problem of explaining that refusing chemotherapy is not tantamount to rejecting the family. So the patient agrees.

Mr Wessels did differ from his fellow patients in that he decided to stop *during* therapy. He did not do this because the therapy was not working, but because he decided that the potential advantages were not worth the disadvantages. In the case of other patients who stopped with therapy it was always the doctor who made the decision, usually because the tumour progressed – continued to grow – during therapy and occasionally for other medical reasons. Many patients complained about the side effects of second- and even third-line therapy, but this never led them to stop.

Biography and development

During the meeting in which Dr Liem revealed that the brain tumour had recurred, Mrs Wessels suddenly realized what the goal of therapy was. I have already described this development in the case of Mr Dekker and later his wife.

I had met Mrs Wessels a year and a half earlier when her husband had been admitted to hospital for tests. The diagnosis was made and he remained in hospital for the first course of treatment. During this period Mrs Wessels was desperate and angry with almost everyone who was involved in her husband's treatment. She thought it was scandalous that they told her so little and she found the ward so filthy that she offered to come and clean it. She often stood in the corridor, upset and ready to attack anyone who passed by. Later she told me that her oldest daughter had died in the Ruysdael Clinic 30 years ago at the age of five. She remembered bringing a child who was mildly ill to the hospital, asking the doctors whether she was getting enough to drink and two weeks later hearing that her child had died, severely dehydrated. She swore never to set foot in the hospital again. When her husband was admitted with a heavy feeling on his chest it was the first time she had been back. How could she trust them to treat her husband properly?

I tell this story to emphasize once again how the biographies of patients and their relatives can determine and explain their actions and attitudes relating to illness. Many considered Mrs Wessels to be a troublesome busybody. The story of her daughter makes her behaviour understandable and makes clear that it was her way of ensuring her husband got proper care. She had never forgiven herself that, 30 years ago, she had not been more insistent that her daughter received more fluid.

Talking about prognosis and variations in the final phase of life

When the hospital can do nothing more for patients in the final phase of their illness they do receive more detailed information about how long they have left and what they can expect from the hospital. The hospital can do nothing more for Mr Wessels because he has refused further therapy. Usually this point is reached when the tumour continues to grow despite therapy, making further treatment pointless. Sometimes the tumour becomes progressive – begins to grow – after a period of remission and cannot be treated. In these cases the doctor tells the patient that nothing more can be done and transfers the patient to the GP. It has become pointless for the patient to continue coming to the hospital. The GP can give the patient all the care necessary for this stage in the illness and trips to the hospital become increasingly difficult as the patient's condition deteriorates. However, if they want, patients can continue to come to the hospital for check-ups.

In this phase doctors usually tell patients that there is not much time remaining and that if they have things to organize they must do that immediately. Sometimes the doctor specifies the time remaining as weeks or, at most, one or two months. If patients or their relatives have questions then the doctor answers these directly. For example, when Mrs Wessels asks Dr Liem how long her husband has left he gives her a relatively detailed answer. He is explicit about the prognosis for the first time.

Dr Liem realizes that Mrs Wessels needs this information and sees that she can cope with it, so he tells her. In their communication doctors respond to patients and their relatives. They try to judge what they want to hear and what they can deal with at that particular time. The pattern of information provision in the case of small-cell lung carcinoma is gradual. They repeat information, gradually adding new details. They interpret questions as expressing a need for information, so the more questions a patient asks the more information the doctor gives. The opposite also applies: if patients do not ask questions then the doctor assumes they do not want to know. As the illness progresses the doctor gives more detailed answers to questions. For example, Dr Liem gave Mrs Wessels a detailed analysis of her husband's prognosis, whereas Dr Heller did not do the same for Mr Wiersema at the start of his second-line therapy.

I also want to mention differences between patients that gradually become visible during treatment and develop into stark contrasts in the final phase. Initially most patients and their relatives react similarly to the initial diagnosis and first-line chemotherapy. They share the same story: the existential crisis followed by adaptation to their illness (see Groen et al. 1995), conscientious compliance to first-line therapy, and hope of cure based on the results of therapy. After the recurrence, during second- and third-line chemotherapy and into the final terminal phase, there is increasing variation. This is a result of both developing coping mechanisms and the course of the illness. Mr Dekker's realization of what was happening developed more rapidly than Mr Wiersema's because the former deteriorated rapidly when his second-line therapy was ineffective, whereas the latter had less serious symptoms because his treatment did work.

Mr and Mrs Wessels said that they experienced the final phase as positive. They were not alone in this. Other couples also experienced it as one of the most beautiful and emotionally intensive periods in their lives.[3] However, as I have mentioned, there was variation, and this will be discussed in Part IV below.

---

3 In an interview in a Dutch weekly (*Vrij Nederland*, 15 January 1998) a widower explains that he considers the final phase of his wife's illness, before she died of lung cancer, as the crown on their marriage.

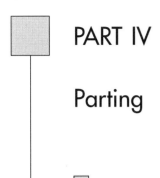

PART IV

Parting

Breaking down optimism and ambivalence

Mr de Jager perseveres

[Ward rounds, 5 September] 'Mr de Jager, born in '36, has been on the ward for two weeks with a small-cell lung carcinoma situated in the right lower lobe, with metastases in the mediastinum' Dr Leo Maas says during the pre-rounds discussion. 'He's had first-line CDE chemotherapy, the last course on the 17th of June. Reported pain two months later, which turned out to be the result of progression. The tumour in the lung increased and a scan revealed metastases in the brain. He's been admitted for second-line chemotherapy. There weren't any neurological symptoms, although he did report reduced sensation in his left leg. But since the 1st of September he's been complaining about loss of power in his legs. So we've requested advice from a neurologist. The patient is to stay in bed until he's seen the neurologist.'

'The neurologist had better come quickly,' says the supervisor. 'A spinal-cord lesion would be catastrophic in this phase. Imagine having to pass your final months like that, crippled and incontinent. There are probably spinal metastases.'

[Ward rounds, 12 September] 'It's become clear that Mr de Jager has multiple spinal metastases, in addition to those in his brain,' Dr Maas reports. The lameness in his legs hasn't improved and he's bedridden. The neurologist will have another look next week. The patient is receiving radiotherapy. The policy is still one of optimal treatment – so no DNR [do not reanimate] order – because of the chemotherapy we've just started. We'll have to await the results of that before deciding further.'

[Ward rounds, 19 September] 'Mr de Jager developed a partial spinal-cord lesion shortly after being admitted, for which he received radiotherapy,' Dr Maas reports. 'He is *leucopenic*, so we've postponed the next course of chemotherapy.

The neurological picture has improved. He can stand up with assistance, but can't walk.'

'He's definitely improved,' says the physiotherapist.

'We have to mobilize him further,' says Dr Maas.

'Has he reached optimal mobilization?' Dr Bron, the supervisor asks the physiotherapist.

'Not by far.'

'Clinical rehabilitation is probably the most useful option, isn't it?' asks Dr Bron.

'Yes,' the physiotherapist says. 'I'm not sure how we would manage that at home, to be honest.'

'What is the situation at home?' the social worker asks.

'He's just moved to a smaller house,' says Dr Maas.

'What's his prognosis?' the social worker asks.

'Poor,' says Dr Maas.

'How poor?'

'Well,' says Dr Bron. 'He's receiving chemotherapy. He could go into remission. It's difficult to say anything about the prognosis. It could take months and it could take years, but he could also deteriorate suddenly.'

'I could discuss with his family about having him home,' the social worker says.

'If we can't send him home then maybe we should think about a nursing home,' says Karel Veenstra, the nurse responsible for Mr de Jager.

'I think that the prognosis is relevant,' the social worker insists. If this is going to be the last time then I think we should do our best. We need to look at all the options. I'll make an appointment with his family.'

[Ward rounds, 30 October] 'Are there any new views on Mr de Jager?' Dr Zorgdrager asks. 'He's been here since the summer.'

'He's very tired these days,' the physiotherapist says. 'But he's said clearly that he wants to continue with rehabilitation.'

'You shouldn't run after him too much,' Dr Zorgdrager says. 'He's in the final stages of a lung carcinoma. We should give him what he wants, no more.' He gets up to look at the X-rays. 'Does everyone know Mr de Jager?' Dr Zorgdrager asks. 'He's a long admittance.'

'And a social problem,' Dr Rutgers sighs.

'I understand he wants to go to a rehabilitation centre,' Dr Zorgdrager says. 'But he doesn't belong in a rehabilitation centre, he belongs in a nursing home.'

'But he *wants* to go to a rehabilitation centre,' the physiotherapist insists.

'Of course,' says Dr Zorgdrager. 'He hopes that they will cure him there. But he doesn't belong there.'

'He says things like that because he doesn't know his own prognosis,' Dr Rutgers says.

'I understand that,' Dr Zorgdrager says. 'But we can't support this request. A nursing home with physiotherapy is better.'

'I understand the choice,' Dr Rutgers says. 'But how do you explain it to him?'

'In a slightly camouflaged way,' Dr Zorgdrager says. Say something like: "You also get physiotherapy in the nursing home, you know".'

'If he knows he only has a few months left he might want to go home,' Theo van Tuuren, one of the nurses, says.

'Precisely. That's exactly how I feel,' Dr Rutgers says. 'Tell him the truth. It's a big shock, but otherwise we're just fooling him.'

'I think he's reached the limit of rehabilitation anyway,' the physiotherapist says.

'Exactly,' says Dr Zorgdrager. That's how we have to present it to him. We say that we're glad that he's made it this far and that we can't get him any better than this.'

'He's concerned about the details,' Theo van Tuuren explains. 'Like being able to walk over to the table from his bed. He doesn't even mention the other issues.'

'So how do we proceed?' Dr Rutgers asks.

'The social worker is going to talk to the family,' Theo van Tuuren says. 'And the family is discussing the situation with the rehabilitation centre.'

Going down fighting

[Ward rounds, 11 December] 'Mr de Jager has been with us a long time,' Dr Mariane Loman, the ward doctor, reports. She summarizes his illness. 'He's being treated with tenoposide,' she continues. 'The last course was postponed for a week because his leucocytes are so low and he's had a fever. Guido Liem gave him the treatment anyway. That was the fifth. We can give him a maximum of 12.

'Damn it,' Dr Bron growls. 'I think it's time we discussed the situation with him. I don't think we should go on like this. This man is going to go down fighting to the bitter end. He's not even halfway through this course of therapy. Let's make another X-ray and see what it looks like locally. Then at least we can determine if there's remission.'

'The neurologist said there was no change,' Dr Loman says.

'That would be something, wouldn't it,' says Dr Bron. 'No change, bad signs in his sputum and fever, all in spite of chemotherapy. When your bone marrow responds like this it's borderline. This is just hopeless.'

'He's waiting for a place in a nursing home.'

'Can he cope mentally?' Dr Bron asks the social worker.

'If he gets into that nursing home, if he gets into that swimming pool,' the social worker says hopelessly.

'He's trying to cope with things by imagining possibilities,' says Dr Bron.

'And he'll keep doing that,' says the social worker. 'Diederik, you keep saying we have to discuss things with him, but are you going to actually do it?'

'Well, err, we'll have to first look at the medical situation objectively and see whether there's a remission or a return of the tumour. If it's the latter then we definitely have to stop with therapy. This man wants to die fighting. That's fine mentally, but he has to be able to cope physically as well, and the therapy is undermining him physically. He can hardly cope with them physically.'

'He thinks things are going to get better once he gets through this phase,' Sanne Wolfensperger, a nurse, says. 'His wife thinks exactly the same way, as though they're investing in the future.'

'I think we have to discuss with the oncologists about the possibility of calling it a day after five or six courses,' Dr Bron says.

'That's difficult, because he knows we can go up to 12, and if we stop early . . .'

'But to go on treating him like that is just delaying the execution,' says Sanne Wolfensperger. 'I think it would be much more acceptable to him if we just told him that his body can't cope with the treatment any more.'

'Yes, we need to have good arguments,' says Dr Bron.

'Mr de Jager is a good example of how things can go wrong'

'I think Mr de Jager is a good example of a case in which discussion of the patient's approaching death was avoided,' says nurse Mirjam Kornelisse. 'He hoped he was going to be cured and those around him confirmed that hope. The longer that went on the more difficult it was to break the illusion. Yet for months the consensus during the pre-rounds discussion was that his interpretation of his chances was totally unrealistic. Mr de Jager is a good example of how it can go wrong. He was given too much hope, by simply not contradicting his own interpretation. It needed one of the doctors to talk to him and break the illusion, but that took a long time to happen. Finally Dr Bron spoke to him and told him clearly that the end was near.

'I think that doctors deprive patients by not telling them the truth. I think that if you tell them the truth it takes a great weight off their shoulders; you give them the chance to say their goodbyes and think about things. After Dr Bron had spoken to him Mr de Jager was a changed man. I talked to him a lot and he accepted that the fight was over. He wanted to spend the time that remained at home doing the things he enjoyed.'

'You mean they had never told him this before?' I ask.

'No,' she shakes her head. 'They tried to say something. For example Dr Zorgdrager had talked to him previously and been quite clear in what he said, but he didn't tell him he was going to die soon. He simply said, "You mustn't expect more progress than there's been up to now. You probably won't be able to do all you can do at the moment. In a wheelchair in the corridor at most. I don't think you'll be able to walk again".'

'How did Mr de Jager react to the news that he was going to die soon?' I ask.

'He seemed to take it in calmly. When I asked him about it later he said that he already knew but was trying to put on a brave face for his wife.'

'I suppose they had to tell him sooner or later,' I say.

'Not sooner or later. They should have told him repeatedly throughout. The problem is that these things are not followed up. The next day the doctor appears at the bedside and pretends all is normal. If you want to do things properly you should have a meeting with the patient and partner at least once a week. Mr de Jager kept some things from his wife, she kept things from him, the doctors didn't tell them everything, and so it goes on. And everyone was aware it was going on. You can avoid that by having regular short meetings in which you discuss things, and not only the medical issues. It needn't take long, 15 minutes or so.

'Talking about death isn't pleasant. I think that's why it's avoided. Here in the hospital we are supposed to treat people, and death doesn't fit into that picture. My husband is a nursing home doctor, and there things are very different. There they take time for discussions like that because it's an integral part of their work. It must be like that for GPs as well. They visit patients every week and talk about coping and that sort of thing. In the hospital how things are done depends a lot on the individual patient. It's that patient who has to take the initiative.'

'How do they tell patients that there's no hope of cure?' I ask.

'You wonder whether that happens early enough. It's not clear right from the start. And you also need to ask yourself whether you are being honest if you offer the patient therapy and say it will extend their life without giving any indication of how long. Is that honest? Can they make a proper choice based on that information?'

'My impression from the discussions is that the important question is *whether* you should tell patients,' I say.

'Yes, I suppose it's difficult to deprive them of all hope,' the nurse says thoughtfully. 'But the question is whether you deprive them of hope by telling them the truth. I'm not sure what the right answer is. I can also see the disadvantages of telling patients directly. I think that quality of life should probably be central. My problem is when I have the feeling that what happens to patients isn't useful. But then, I'm not a doctor, so I can't really judge. I had an experience recently. When patients are offered chemotherapy I often think, "Is that really necessary?" Mr Bokjes, for example. Such a small, frail man, who ended up on the ward in a dip after every course of treatment. I really thought, "What are we doing to him?" One day I saw him in the X-ray department. He told me that things were fine and that he'd had a very pleasant summer. Then I thought to myself, "Well, maybe it's a good thing he had that chemotherapy after all."'

'The best strategy is probably to decide for each individual patient. But that's also difficult. We nurses often *think* we know a lot about the patients. A patient has hardly arrived on the ward and we already know the situation,' She smiles. 'I sometimes wonder what makes us so certain that we know it all. But then, the doctors don't see the patients that much themselves. They see them mainly on paper and X-rays. So how can you determine what's best for the patient? You do it on the basis of the facts you have, but it isn't a very sound one. Unless the patient has been on the ward for months it remains guesswork to some extent.'

'They never contradict us'

Jantien Mulder enters the doctor's consulting room alone and takes a seat opposite Dr Liem. 'My father doesn't want to come to the hospital anymore,' she explains. 'I tried to persuade him but he was adamant. He doesn't want anything anymore. But I have a few questions, which is why I've come instead.' Her tone is businesslike, but not unfriendly.

'You've been on holiday,' she continues. 'And in your absence all kinds of things have happened. My father became very confused. He imagined himself to be in the strangest places, and it become untenable. He was admitted to hospital and diagnosed with brain metastases. The gave him dexametason and radiotherapy.'

Dr Liem nods. 'I've heard from the neurologist,' he says.

'He responded well to the treatment and his condition improved greatly. At home he regained an interest in things and was jolly. He had a good time. And to be honest with you, we began to silently hope that something more might be possible. But now, less than two months later, he's collapsed again.' Her eyes become moist and she swallows. 'We've been told things. We spoke to the ward doctor in neurology. First they said that things were bad, and then they said that things were improving. What should we expect? It's not clear to us at all. When my father seemed to recover we told the neurologist that we were starting to have hope, and that wasn't contradicted. They let us talk like that, which made us think that maybe he had a future.' Dr Liem nods understandingly. He respects people who address the issues directly. 'Everyone in the hospital is busy,' Jantien Mulder continues. 'I can understand that. I'm also busy at work. For the doctors and nurses I'm simply Mr Mulder's daughter. But he is not just a case for me, he's my father.'

'Your father had a problem with his shoulder,' Dr Liem says. 'We weren't sure whether the tumour had developed further or whether there were metastases. It turned out to be the latter. The cancer had spread through the blood, which made his prognosis worse, because if the cancer cells are in the blood then they can be anywhere in the body. Then he was diagnosed with brain metastases, which made his prognosis even worse. That means he doesn't have much time left.'

'Not much time,' she repeats.

'You have to think in terms of months, if not weeks,' Dr Liem continues. Tears stream over her cheeks. She takes a handkerchief from her bag and wipes her eyes. 'Sorry,' she says. 'I didn't mean to . . .' She smiles sadly at Dr Liem. 'He'd so hoped . . .'

'I'm sorry,' says Dr Liem.

'It can't be helped,' she says.

'It sounds hard,' Dr Liem says. 'But it's better that you know. It's better for your father as well.'

She nods. 'That's what I'm here for.'

'That means,' Dr Liem continues, 'that if there are things that need arranging then you must do that now. It would also be good for him to know what he can expect from the hospital. To be honest, that isn't much. I think that in this phase your father is better off at home than here between all the white coats.'

'Yes,' she says.

'Listen, if there was something we could do for him then we would do it. But there isn't, so it's better for him to stay at home and be looked after there. His GP can do as much for him as we can, perhaps more. He should try to make your father's remaining time as pleasant as possible.'

Jantien Mulder says she is happy now that she knows the truth. 'All that avoidance makes it difficult,' she says. 'I can understand it, but it makes it difficult for us. And things have gone really fast. It's less than a year ago that we sat here looking at that first scan, when you explained what the problem was. I'll never forget that moment.' She stares at the floor. 'Anyway, in a car crash you're gone even quicker.' Dr Liem smiles. 'Our family is small,' she continues, 'only a brother, my mother and an old granny. That's all. Ach,' she says, putting her hand before her mouth. 'You're not interested in that. So there's no need for us to come back to the hospital?'

'No. I'd cancel all further appointments,' Dr Liem confirms. 'I'll phone the GP and inform him of this conversation.' Jantien Mulder stands up. 'Thank you,' she says as she shakes Dr Liem's hand.

Practical explanations

When patients are undergoing first-line chemotherapy and in the subsequent period of recovery their optimism is understandable. In Chapter 5 I argued that it is difficult for patients to interpret the changes on the X-rays and the doctors' positive comments in any other way. The effect of chemotherapy *resembles* cure (The et al. 1996a). But optimism in that phase of the illness also has a function. One can argue whether or not it is good for patients to hold on to a belief that turns out to be an illusion, but everyone agrees that it is the hope of a cure that gives patients and their relatives the strength to carry on and to endure treatment.[1]

However, in the phase of the illness in which Mr de Jager finds himself, optimism about recovery is totally misplaced. Here it was not only the nurses who were critical of his optimism; it made everyone who was involved in his treatment nervous. His condition was deteriorating rapidly and it was clear to all that he did not have long to go, but in spite of this he struggled against the tide, anticipating the day when he could pick up the threads of his normal life again. It became embarrassing to observe the doctors and nurses silently listening to his announcements about rehabilitation.

---

1 See for example the reflection of the patients' widows in Chapter 12.

For months his totally misplaced interpretation of his situation was the subject of discussion before ward rounds, and the doctors wrestled with the question of whether or not they should break down his false hopes. They discussed this dilemma endlessly behind the closed doors of their office but hardly at all with the patient himself. The odd doctor tried subtly to change Mr de Jager's mind, but in vain. When these attempts failed, they were abandoned.

To some extent this chain of events is a product of the practical factors inherent in the kind of hospital that the Ruysdael Clinic was; a large teaching hospital. When I studied my notes later I was struck by the number of doctors who had been involved in his case while he was on the ward. He had been there during the summer, during which time many of the doctors had gone on leave. This, combined with changing shifts meant that there was a rapid turnover in junior ward doctors and, to a lesser extent, supervisors (and in my presentation I have reduced the number of doctors to make it easier for the reader to follow). These changes tended to exacerbate communication difficulties between those involved.

Codes of conduct also play a role: locums will attempt to interfere as little as possible with the general policy of the doctor they are replacing, and they will tend not to provide different kinds of information to the patient either. But there are also practical reasons. Being temporarily involved with a patient, it is difficult to know what information colleagues have already provided. Active involvement is also rather pointless because they cannot really contribute to the longer-term process of information provision. This was not necessarily experienced as a problem; some were thankful to be spared having to solve these complex problems. Cases like that of Mr de Jager do not stem only from the changing shifts of doctors and there were other patients in the same situation. Indeed, nurses regularly complained about doctors 'passing the buck'.

Doctors and the dilemma of optimism

The reason doctors gave for being careful about what they told Mr de Jager was that they were not sure that confronting him with the truth would have helped him. During discussions, both on the ward and in the outpatient clinic, a recurring theme was whether doctors should take away patients' last hopes by imposing the truth on them. Individual doctors had different opinions on this, which related to the previously mentioned styles of practice.

On the ward Dr Bron was a doctor who avoided confronting patients with the hard truth. He introduced the topic carefully and if the patient did not respond then he did not insist. Maarten Rutgers and Ilona Racz preferred to give patients a clear picture of their situation right from the start. They were of the opinion that the illusion of recovery does not spare patients. They thought it better to tell them the truth, even if this came as a blow, so that they could then learn to live with it. Not telling patients the truth deprives them of the possibility of rounding off their lives and saying goodbye, and it is much more difficult for them to cope with the truth later when they find out anyway.

The doctors in the outpatient clinic had an approach similar to that of Dr Bron, and they did not make much effort to relieve patients of their hope of cure. However, this did change in the final phase of the patient's life, and Dr Liem in particular would take the initiative and explain the situation to patients. His interviews with Mr and Mrs Wessels and Jantien Mulder are good examples of this. Dr Liem felt that patients had a right to this knowledge in the final weeks of life so that they can make their final preparations. There was therefore a transition in the final phase of Dr Liem's process of gradual information provision, and this was a conscious strategy on his part. At that point he felt that it had become necessary to break down the patient's hope. The pattern of information provision used by Dr Ronald Veerman was very similar, although in his case the final transition was less pronounced.

In the case of Dr Heller there was hardly any change in information provision in the final phase. I do not think this has to do with him having a different vision or strategy but rather with the fact that he simply found it difficult to give patients bad news. It sometimes seemed as though he wanted to tell them but was not sure how to. The final meeting with Mr Dekker, which I describe in Chapter 12, is a good example of this.

The discussion above gives the impression that the hope of cure can only be broken down by doctors informing patients about the truth of their situation, and that the source of hope lies exclusively in what doctors tell patients. The cases of Mr de Jager and Mr Mulder illustrate that hope also springs from what doctors *do not say* and from what patients and their relatives say that doctors *do not contradict*. Mr Mulder and his family interpreted the doctor's silence as a confirmation of their statements, as a positive sign. Because patients' expectations and plans are not contradicted their hope of cure is given space to develop.

The doctors' reasons for silence in the case of Mr Mulder were different from those in the case of Mr de Jager. I have already explained that it is the task of the specialist in charge to determine the general policy toward a patient, and the lung specialists were in charge of both men's treatment. However, Mr de Jager was a patient in the Lung Department whereas Mr Mulder ended up in the Neurology Department, being treated by neurologists who were ultimately not responsible for providing him with general information about his prognosis. This was similar to Mrs Dekker's position in the Radiology Department. In Chapter 8, I described how the radiologist made it clear to Mrs Dekker that she could not tell her anything and that she should ask the lung specialist in charge of her husband's treatment.

However, it is not only what doctors do and do not say that inspires hope. Hope springs from the very presence of doctors and their technical arsenal (Tannen 1993). In Chapter 8 the nurse Carola Vroom remarked how difficult it was for patients to refuse the treatment that has been offered. This is even true in cases where it has been made clear to the patient that the treatment will have no therapeutic effect.[2] When patients agree to therapy their reasoning is, 'You never know, it might help'. The very idea that they are undergoing treatment gives them hope.

Doctors also give patients hope against their own better judgement, however. This stems from various factors, including the doctors' medical training. For example, until not so long ago medical students in the Netherlands were taught that they should not allow patients to lose hope, even when they were terminally ill. But they also include such things as lack of time and nerve. I remarked earlier that doctors use the argument that they are doing 'what is good for the patient' to justify holding back. It is also emotionally very difficult for a doctor to dash the hope of a patient who desperately wants to get better.[3] Emotions have a resonating effect. Seeing someone laugh makes you want to laugh as well, even though you do not know what they are laughing about. Seeing a sad or despondent patient makes one sad and despondent; seeing someone suffer can be painful. Moreover, the mortality of patients confronts doctors with their own mortality. It is this resonance that can make working in the health sector so difficult (see also The 1997a, Chapter 1).

Nurses sometimes criticize doctors for avoiding discussion of death. Many of them thought that doctors should be much more forceful in cases such as that of Mr de Jager, that they should have broken down his hope and made him face the facts. Mirjam Kornelisse expressed what nurses saw as the solution: spend more time on the bad news interview and keep coming back to it afterwards. Their view is that bad news needs to be repeated.

Finally I would like to mention the way in which Mr Mulder's daughter talked to Dr Liem. She approached the doctor in exactly the right way, not reproachful or emotional but direct and almost business-like. In return she receives a direct and honest answer. I do not want to suggest that Jantien Mulder only received an honest answer because of her conversational style, however. The fact that Mr Mulder was in the very final phase of his illness also played a role. In Chapter 7, I noted that patients and their relatives often assume they do not have a right to occupy the doctor's time with private matters. Jantien Mulder was no exception. She apologized when she cried and when she explained the family situation. Her tone was not exclusively apologetic, though, and there was some irony as well, as though she wanted to show that she was aware of the relationships in the hospital.

---

2 For example in Phase 1 trials. See also Brinkman-Woltjer et al. (1988).
3 I have personally experienced just how difficult this is.

Two sides to the story

'I think doctors are good at *curing*, and in those situations doctors and nurses collaborate well,' says René Hartog. He is perched on the edge of his chair. We have been talking for more than half an hour and he is becoming increasingly enthralled by his own exposition. 'But when it comes to *care*', he continues, 'they're often nowhere to be seen and we nurses have to cope alone. Then you have to be direct, asking them things, demanding that they take action. Doctors are focused on patients getting better, but that doesn't always happen; sometimes they don't get better and they die. I think that when a patient is going to die you have to make it as easy as possible; and we can do that, we have the means. My impression is that doctors are scared to do that, and scared of each other. Haven't you noticed how they procrastinate? They're scared of criticism from senior colleagues; worried it might influence their career prospects.

'Patients come to hospital to get better. In fact, dying doesn't really belong in a hospital. It's understandable. Doctors want to shine with successfully cured patients. They want to be God. It's pleasant to be seen as a *healer*. When the average survival time is five years, doctors talk about cure. They give chemotherapy, but the tumour always recurs, and patients suffer the side effects of treatment; they spend their final months feeling sick and weak in the hospital.

'Of course, I realize that there are two sides to this; the patient also plays a role, clinging to life right to the end, clutching at every straw. And that helps to keep medicine on its pedestal. Doctors are able to see themselves as gods because of the expectations of those who are dependent on them. If the patients, the consumers, realized what they were letting themselves in for then I'm not so sure whether they would make that choice. Because it's also possible to do nothing, just give pain-relief medication. Perhaps the patient can still spend some weeks, maybe months, at home before dying. All this treatment makes health care so expensive. And with what result? Maybe we should rethink our priorities and only give palliative care.

'The results of treatment in patients I've seen treated for cancer are relative, hardly ever great. Maybe they live for a few months longer, but those months are often dreadful. Patients are obsessed with treatment because that's what they've been taught. Medicine has presented itself as heroic. They've seen successful heart transplants, bypass surgery, you name it. They've seen successful treatment.'

The Riddle, the medics and society

Nuland describes how, as a child, he admired his family's calm, confidence-inspiring doctor, and how this influenced his ambition to become a doctor. During his medical training, however, he realized that to really count in the profession, solving *The Riddle* was often more important than the welfare of individual patients. Diagnosis and technical solutions were what medicine was all about. Nuland argues that doctors can solve *The Riddle* by clinical action, while at the same time losing the struggle for humane patient care. He claims that there are few specialists who can claim that they have never persuaded patients to accept diagnostic and therapeutic interventions on such unreasonable grounds that it would have been better to leave *The Riddle* unsolved.

> Too often near the end, were the doctor able to see deeply within himself, he might recognize that his decisions and advice are motivated by his inability to give up *The Riddle* and admit defeat as long as there is any chance of solving it, Though he be kind and considerate of the patient he treats, he allows himself to push his kindness aside because the seduction of *The Riddle* is so strong and the failure to solve it renders him so weak.
>
> Nuland (1995: 249)

One of the reasons, noted by both Nuland and René Hartog, that doctors persevere with tests and treatment is the fear of criticism by colleagues. Doctors also want to be healers.

The story of patients' hope is more complex, however. René Hartog touches on another factor: the heroic presentation of medicine in relation to which patients' expectations have developed. In our society, the narratives that are presented publicly are recovery narratives (Frank 1995). Patients have only been exposed to success stories, so it is hardly surprising that their expectations of what medicine can do are often (too) high. During my study, one of the lung oncologists participated in a television programme about lung cancer. A patient was filmed undergoing surgery. The idea was that the patient would be interviewed when he was better, six months after the operation. Unfortunately the patient died, so another one was recruited for the post-operative interview. I could give many more examples. In television soap series patients are shown recovering from major life-threatening illnesses as though it were the most normal thing in the world. In spite of the odd scandal, doctors are still generally presented as heroes in the media. The picture of medical success is also maintained partly because that is what people want. Doctors are influenced by society and express a social desire to deny death. Even if they wanted to, it would be difficult for doctors to do otherwise.

'Do I have to repeat it again?'

Dr Liem is not looking forward to the next consultation. He pages through the file, buttons his white coat, drums his fingers on the table, drains the last drop of coffee from the plastic cup and flicks it in the waste paper basket. He sighs. 'These people are deeply disappointed,' he says. I look up questioningly. 'Mr Aalders has had chemotherapy,' he explains. 'Then after a while he developed metastases in the brain. He's receiving radiotherapy. The news of the metastases hit them like a bomb. It was a terrible disappointment. They just can't understand how it is possible. They were here last week and I tried to explain things to them carefully, but they were very emotional. It was very difficult, so I asked them to come back today.' He gets up from his chair and goes out to the waiting room, returning a moment later with Mr and Mrs Aalders.

Mr Aalders says things are fine. The lameness that was the first sign of the brain metastases has disappeared. But they do have a burning question. 'If it comes back . . .' Mr Aalders begins, shifting about on the edge of his chair. 'If it comes back, will I be able to have radiotherapy again, doctor?' He chews nervously on his gum. Beads of sweat are visible on his forehead.

'That's the problem with this tumour,' Dr Liem says quietly. 'If it does come back then we can't give you radiotherapy again, not to your head.'

'Oh my God,' cries Mrs Aalders.

'We understood that you said that it was possible,' Mr Aalders says. 'You said ten times, then after that another ten times.'

'Yes, if the cancer reappears somewhere else then we can do it again,' Dr Liem explains. 'But not if it comes back in the same place.'

'Well, that's how we interpreted it,' Mr Aalders says. 'Ten times, then we'd see how things looked, then another ten times.'

'Well, they might have some new programme in Radiotherapy that I'm unaware of,' Dr Liem says. 'You'd have to ask them.'

'Yes well, that's how we interpreted it,' Mr Aalders repeats. Silence falls.

'It's a difficult question,' Dr Liem says after a while. I notice that he emphasizes the words. 'But I must say that, generally speaking, the answer to your question is "no". Radiotherapy in the same spot is not possible. If the tumour reappears elsewhere then we'll have to see what can be done. But the more often it comes back, the more difficult it's going to be to treat it.'

'Phew!' exclaims Dr Liem when he has closed the door behind Mr and Mrs Aalders. 'I find that really difficult. I'm not sure exactly what to say. Just before the radiotherapy I told them that his life expectation was very low. They both cried terribly. What else can I do? Do I have to repeat it again? They looked much better than on previous occasions. Should I go and sour things by being honest again, by telling them things I've already told them? It's a real problem.'

'He could have persevered with his questioning,' I say. 'He didn't ask how long he still had left.'

'Precisely,' says Dr Liem. 'That's exactly what I mean. I tell them once or twice what the situation is. If they want to know more they can ask. I leave it to them.'

'Do you find it difficult to pass on such bad news?'

'Not for myself. I think they have a right to know what their position is. But it's difficult for them. What damage do I do with my words? That's my problem.'

Mrs Gruter gets better

Mrs Gruter has laid her head on the table and cries loudly. 'Oh,' she cries. 'How is this possible? How could this happen?' Her husband is next to her. He has put his arm round her. His glasses are on the table. Their daughter has moved around to the back of Mrs Gruter's chair and is holding her mother tightly. Dr Liem looks on helplessly. 'I can imagine that this news has hit you hard,' he says, trying to resume the conversation. Mrs Gruter's hopeless moaning continues. 'Quiet now mum,' the daughter says, looking apologetically at Dr Liem. I see him searching for the right words. Then he picks up his pen and writes, 'diagnosis: small-cell lung carcinoma, extensive disease with liver metastases. Patient informed about the advantages and disadvantages of therapy. She has decided to accept CDE chemotherapy.' Dr Liem tries to concentrate on what he is writing, occasionally stealing a glance at Mrs Gruter.

'How's it possible? How did I get this,' Mrs Gruter howls.

'Yes, it's unpleasant,' Dr Liem mumbles.

'I've always worked hard, I brought up seven children. I haven't done anything wrong, have I?'

Two weeks later Dr Liem hangs up the X-rays. 'I'll show you what's happened,' he says. Mr and Mrs Gruter are standing next to him, holding hands. 'Look here,' Dr Liem says. 'This is the X-ray made before treatment. Here you can see a large tumour. Then here we have the X-ray that was made today. Do you see the difference?'

'Oh!' Mrs Gruter exclaims. 'It's almost gone.'

'Yes,' Dr Liem smiles. 'The tumour has reduced significantly. It's hardly visible. The treatment has had an effect.'

'Oh, it's almost disappeared,' says Mrs Gruter, starting to cry. 'It's wonderful. Look, it's almost completely disappeared.' Her husband embraces her. 'Oh doctor, I'm so happy.'

'Yes, it's a good result, after three courses of therapy,' Dr Liem says.

Another two weeks later I am in Dr Liem's office. 'Great stuff!' he exclaims, clapping his hands happily. 'Complete remission.'

'Mrs Gruter?' I ask.

'Yes. I'll call them in and tell them.'

'Nice to give some good news for a change?'

'Certainly,' he says as he strides confidently into the waiting room.

'How are things?' he asks Mrs Gruter a few minutes later when they are all seated in his office. She gives him a thumbs-up sign. 'I can do everything again, all the housework, riding my bicycle.' Her husband nods.

'Great,' Dr Liem says. 'And I've got good news for you.' He gets up and walks over to the X-rays. 'You've had your last course of therapy and now we need to take stock. Here are all the X-rays, the first one at the start, in the middle of treatment and then the most recent one made today. You can see how the tumour rapidly shrank and now . . . Well . . .' He leans forward. 'There's some slight marking just here, but I can only see that because I know you. If I hadn't known I wouldn't have noticed anything.'

'I'm better!' Mrs Gruter exclaims, leaning on her husband and weeping. 'I'm cured! Oh I had so hoped.'

'Well, we need to wait and see *what* happens next,' Dr Liem says, leaving a silence for the words to sink in. 'But at the moment, things look fine.'

Subsequent check-up visits are almost identical. Dr Liem asks how things are; Mrs Gruter gives him a thumbs-up; Dr Liem tells her the situation is 'stable' or 'unchanged'; the tears flow – tears of happiness, she explains. At the end of every consultation she says, 'I am completely better, aren't I, doctor?' The first few times she asks this Dr Liem shifts about nervously and tries to break the illusion; later he hardly responds. In the waiting room I often chat with Mr and Mrs Gruter. 'That doctor,' she says repeatedly, shaking her head. 'That doctor is like this,' and she gives her habitual thumbs-up. 'He makes me so happy I could throw my arms round him and hug him.'

One day Mrs Gruter is going through the usual motions of telling us how good she feels. Today, however, Dr Liem's face is grim. 'I have the latest X-rays,' he interrupts her calmly but urgently. His tone shocks her. 'I'm afraid the tumour has reappeared,' he says. 'Look, here is the X-ray from your last visit, and here is today's.' A white patch is clearly visible on the latter. There can be no doubt. Mrs Gruter buries her face in her hands and begins to tremble. She gradually becomes more emotional, and her husband begins to cry.

'Very unpleasant, very unpleasant,' says Dr Liem. 'We need to discuss what we're going to do. I think you should resume chemotherapy as soon as possible.' The Gruters both nod. 'Preferably immediately, after this meeting,' Dr Liem continues. They nod again. 'Do you agree?' Dr Liem asks. More nodding. Dr Liem takes an application form and starts to fill it in.

It is three weeks later. Mr and Mrs Gruter stand hand-in-hand in front of the most recent X-rays. She has completed the first course of treatment and Dr Liem is showing then how the tumour has again reduced in size.

'Yes, I can see it's become smaller,' Mrs Gruter says.

'The chemotherapy has worked again,' Dr Liem says. He sounds relieved. Mrs Gruter cries. 'It's a good result,' says Dr Liem.

History repeats itself. The tumour gradually shrinks. Mrs Gruter feels great, she can cope with the housework again. She weeps whenever Dr Liem says he is satisfied. 'Oh doctor, I'm so happy,' she says, looking admiringly at Dr Liem. 'I'm getting better,' she tells her husband. 'The doctor's making me better again, do you hear?' Mr Gruter nods emotionally. Then one day, at the end of a consultation she says, 'Doctor, I've got a question. Will you help me if it goes wrong again?'

'We'll have to analyse the situation when the time comes. There are possibilities, but it will get more difficult. The fact that the tumour has returned already makes it more difficult to treat you.'

'So you will help?'

'We've still got various options.'
'You hear that?' she asks her husband. 'The doctor is going to help me again.'
She dabs her eyes with a tissue. 'The tumour has gone again, but for how long?
Last time it disappeared, but it came back again.'
'That's the question,' Dr Liem says, raising his arms in the air. 'We'll just have
to wait and see.'
'So it will come back?' Mr Gruter mumbles.
'Yes.'
'Again and again?'
'Again and again.'
'Until . . . ?'
'Until there's nothing more we can do.'
'Until the end?'
'Yes.'
'Did you hear that,' Mrs Gruter exclaims. 'Dr Liem is going to help me. I'm so
happy.'
'Come on,' Dr Liem says to me wearily after they have left. 'I need some coffee.'
'Mr Gruter realizes what the situation is,' I say while Dr Liem pours the coffee.
'Yes, he knows.'
'I think she also knows,' I add. Dr Liem nods.
'She does now,' he says. 'At first I tried to make it clear to her, but did you see
how she responded?'
'Yes, she was getting better.'
'Exactly.' Dr Liem sips his coffee. 'So I just left it that way. It's rather pointless
trying to break through that optimism and force them to see the truth.'
'She said she was getting better again today,' I say. 'But at the same time she
wanted to know whether you'd help her again next time. I interpreted that as a
sign that she knew what was coming. But she is ambiguous.'
'That's often the case. I used to find that really difficult. I once had a patient
with lung cancer. He'd been treated a number of times and I told him that
he didn't have long to go. The next day during rounds he looked so jolly, I
wondered whether he'd understood what I'd told him. So I went over and talked
to him, explained his situation again. He was discharged and then admitted
again shortly after. Still very jolly. Told me about holiday plans. Again I wondered whether he understood, so I started explaining once more. He interrupted
me. "Doctor," he said. "You told me this when I was first diagnosed with cancer,
then you told me again when the tumour recurred. Now you're telling me for the
third time. I've got the message, you know." That really put me in my place.'

Patients' ambivalence

René Hartog claims that patients are also responsible for the narrative of
hope. During my study I noticed that whenever a patient did not know

or understand something, whether in a bad news interview or relating to informed consent, it was always the doctor's fault. Here I do not intend to judge doctors' communicative skills, but shifting all responsibility onto the doctors does seem to be rather simplistic, as this would imply that it is only they who have the power to give or take away hope. Patients want to get better and they construct their world around that desire. When patients do not want to hear that they will not get better, then they do not hear it.

Dr Liem sounded tired when he said, 'I tell them but it doesn't come across,' after the consultation with Mr Aalders. I often heard doctors talk like this. Dr Veerman said that at the start of his career he sometimes doubted whether he had given patients information in the right way. He hesitated to find fault with the patient so he blamed himself. Until he over-heard a patient, on whom he had just spent three-quarters of an hour explaining what was wrong with him, saying to another patient, 'You don't get much information from the doctors do you? They never tell you what's wrong with you'. This was so far from the truth that Dr Veerman suddenly realized that the fault was not always on his side. He realized that, in this case at least, there was an independent and capricious variable that he could not control. Dr Veerman made use of a code. At the start of the illness he tells patients what is wrong with them twice. After that he answers questions, no more. He only volunteers information about their condition when it becomes necessary, when there is a recurrence.

It can easily be forgotten that these doctors are confronted with seriously ill patients who want to get better. They and their relatives are ready to clutch at any straw, whether this is therapy options or doctors' statements that they have misinterpreted. As a result they find themselves in a mael-strom of medical last resorts. They agree to these because they interpret them as more hopeful than they actually are. In this way patients and their relatives attempt to deny approaching death. However doctors present their message, patients must want to hear it. It is only when they are emotionally ready that they can properly interpret what the doctor is saying. As I have already commented this is a gradual development that cannot be forced.

More is involved, however. What, for example, should we make of Dr Liem's optimistic patient, making plans as though he was unaware that he would not be there to see them through, but in fact well aware of his situation? Part of the problem was that the patient did not behave in a way that doctors and nurses expected of someone who was dying. If he had spoken about his condition, been sad, or angry, then this misunder-standing would not have arisen. Perhaps he simply enjoyed making plans. Should patients be deprived of that because they are dying? The same reasoning could be applied to the hope of cure. They might know that they are going to die but the will to live is so strong that they hope against all odds that a miracle will happen. During my study I noticed that the realiza-tion of approaching death is latent (Sheehy 1973). Whether it is expressed or masked by hope depends on the situation (Marshal 1980: 138). It is possible that this is what was happening in the case of Mrs Gruter, that she knew that she was going to die while at the same time believing that she was getting better. The same might apply to Mr de Jager, who told the nurse that he knew he was dying but wanted to keep this from his wife, and to Mrs Wessels, who described how she knew and at the same time did not know that her husband had a fatal illness; how the realization of what the doctors really meant dawned on her during the final stage of his illness. Because of the complexity of psychological defence mechanisms it is difficult to be certain about the exact extent of this realization (Kellehear 1992: 75).

11 The familiar hospital

Mr and Mrs Wessels keep coming to the outpatient clinic

Mr Wessels completes second-line chemotherapy in October. The family celebrates his birthday in November with an Indonesian meal. They enjoy Christmas together. The grandchildren come and stay during the spring holiday, and his brother comes over from Australia at Easter. Mr Wessels passes away, against all expectations, after Whitsuntide.

Throughout this period he still faithfully attends the outpatient clinic, carried in on a trolley. He waits patiently in a separate room down the corridor until one of the doctors has time to see him. As they wait, he and his wife chat to the nurses, fellow patients and me. He says it is 'nice' to come to the hospital; at least he can be himself there. Unlike Mrs Wessels, who asks everyone for advice about how to take care of her husband, Mr Wessels hardly mentions his illness except to crack cynical jokes with Mark van Rossum, his favourite nurse, about his approaching end. Friends and relatives at home do not see the humour of these jokes, so he saves them for the hospital.

Mrs Wessels says that they have become attached to the outpatient clinic and the staff during the 18 months that they have been coming. Rather than consulting their GP, she prefers to discuss problems with Dr Liem, even though it is time-consuming coming in to the hospital from the village where they live. She does not get on well with the GP. She thinks that he did not interpret her husband's early symptoms properly and as a result referred him to the hospital too late. She prefers Dr Liem and the hospital. And she always has a lot of questions. Dr Liem tells me that she also phones him a few times a week, sometimes daily, with questions. In the weekends, when Dr Liem is not available, Mrs Wessels turns to me as a stand-in. Mrs Wessels's phone calls became a regular feature of my early Sunday mornings. One morning I enter Dr Liem's office. He puts his pen down and looks at me. I greet him. 'I've been speaking to Mrs Wessels,' he says and falls silent, looking at me critically. Oh God, I think. I haven't told him I've been speaking to her on the phone. I might have been giving her the wrong advice. 'Yes,' he continues, with the hint of a smile. 'I gather that we're sharing the care of this patient, and that you're guaranteeing that I have a bit of free time in my weekends.'

Attachment and parting

I ask Mark van Rossum what he thinks about Mr and Mrs Wessels still coming in to the hospital.

'It happens a lot,' he answers. 'When I hear that they have an appointment six weeks or three months later then I know what the situation is. They either have an untreatable recurrence or they've stopped treatment altogether, like Mr Wessels. The hospital can't help them anymore and they've usually been told as much. But if they're still alive then most of them still come in for their appointment. And when I ask them why, they say it's for the recognition and to see us all.'

'You've gone through a lot together,' I say.

'Yes, good times and bad times. Our involvement is intensive but varied. We're there right from the start, and when the end comes, I must admit, it sometimes affects me. I try to keep a professional distance, but I don't always succeed. When René Hartog died, for example, I thought it was terrible. I got on really well with him and his wife, Linda. You try to be professional, but you can't always avoid that side of things. You meet so many people, and with some of them you get on so well that in another context you'd become friends. When they die, it touches you. Mr van der Velden, René Hartog, Brigit Westra, they were special people; I didn't want them to die.

'Do you keep in touch with the partner afterwards?' I ask.

'In some cases I quite consciously say goodbye. I often represent the department at the funeral, to achieve some sort of closure. It's good for me, for them and for us here in the hospital. I kept in touch with René Hartog's wife. That peters out after a while, but that's okay.'

'I've never heard of doctors doing that.'

'Seldom, but it also depends on the doctor. Dorien Meulman, for example, is very different from the lung specialists. She went much further in her contact with patients, and she showed emotion. There are patients who specifically request her because they can talk to her. She's not scared to present herself as vulnerable. When René said goodbye, Dorien and I cried. Guido, Marcel and Ronald have more of a doctor–patient relationship. But patients don't always see that as negative. They like Guido Liem, for example, even though he has the reputation for keeping his distance. Maybe it's a conscious strategy on the part of the doctors, otherwise they wouldn't be able to function. Maybe they decide to go that far and no further.

'I think that emotions are part of our work. If I didn't have them and couldn't show them, then that would be a bad sign. But it remains work, and you shouldn't lose sight of that either. I've managed to strike a balance over the years.'

Mr Fresco goes home

The 47-year-old Mr Carlos Fresco occupies a single room on the ward. He participated in the same trial as Mr Wiersema and Mr Dekker. He was seriously confused and was admitted two days ago. He is agitated and prowls the corridors at night, a packet of tobacco in hand, looking for somewhere to smoke. During the day he cannot sit still and keeps threatening to run away. The nurses have their hands full. Sanne Wolfensperger, the social worker, is consulted. She spends the better part of a morning with him. Mr Fresco is receiving second-line chemotherapy. He is on the third course. During rounds it becomes apparent that there is progression in spite of the therapy. His confusion suggests further development of the brain metastases that were the first sign of a recurrence. 'We can't do anything more for this man,' says Dr Bron. 'It's a question of weeks, more likely days. Radiotherapy might be an option, though.'

In the afternoon Mr Fresco's GP contacts the ward doctor. He wants to know the details of Mr Fresco's brain metastases. He thinks they should send Mr Fresco home before it is too late. He also thinks radiotherapy is a bad idea. 'This man isn't very intelligent to start with. If you give him radiotherapy he's going to end up as an imbecile. I think he should be allowed to die peacefully, preferably at home,' the GP says. He has come to the hospital to see his patient, but Mr Fresco is nowhere to be found. He leaves a note on his bed. On his way out he sees Mr Fresco sitting among the large potted plants with his head in his hands. The GP kneels next to him and puts a hand on his shoulder. Later I ask Mr Fresco what he discussed with the GP. 'About me going home as soon as possible,' he says.

That afternoon there is a meeting. Mr Fresco's small room is full: Mr Fresco, his brother and sister, his partner and her daughter, Dr Veerman, Dr Terpstra, Alexandra Visser (one of the nurses) and Sanne Wolfensperger (the social worker). Mr Fresco's relatives and the girlfriend do not appear to be on good terms. Dr Veerman explains the situation. It is a hopeless situation. They cannot do anything more for Mr Fresco in the hospital. This is a hard blow for the partner and she bursts into tears.

'Is there really nothing you can do?' she pleads.

Dr Veerman shakes his head. 'We've done everything we can,' he says.

'I knew there was something wrong,' the sister says. 'But you,' she says spitefully to Mr Fresco's partner. 'You don't want to admit it to yourself. Whenever there's anything unpleasant, you just shut your eyes.'

Dr Veerman starts talking about sending Mr Fresco home. He explains to the family that this depends on them. The sister says she promised her mother to look

after her little brother come what may, and she is ready to do all that is necessary. The partner objects. She cannot spend the night with Mr Fresco because
she is worried they might cut her Social Security benefit. She lives far away from
his house and will not be able to get a bus home every evening. So the discussion goes on. Dr Veerman and Dr Terpstra leave the room. Mr Fresco gets up
and wants to go home immediately. Alexandra is on the phone trying to arrange
home care. I escort the emotional partner and her daughter to another room.
There the crying degenerates into a diatribe against Mr Fresco's relatives: they
are vultures after his money. The brother has to go to work and leaves. The sister
goes and sits in the corridor, ready to take Mr Fresco home. Mr Fresco stumbles
up and down the corridor, not sure who to go to. He finds his partner and sees
she is crying.

'What's wrong?' he asks.

'Nothing,' she says.

Mr Fresco goes back to his sister. The social worker joins them. She promises
to visit them at home. She says they can call her if there is a problem. Everyone
is happy about that.

Mr Fresco's partner sends him to the hospital

A week later Mr Fresco's partner steers him into the outpatient clinic in a
wheelchair. He is so confused he hardly knows where he is. The people in the
waiting room are moved. Dr Veerman is busy and asks Dr Heller if he can see
Mr Fresco straight away. He explains that Mr Fresco was discharged two weeks
previously, that there was nothing more they could do for him and that his family
was aware of the situation. 'The problem is,' he continues, 'that they're rather
attached to the hospital. There's no need to examine him, there's nothing you
can do, just see them and talk to them. In fact, it's a miracle he's still alive.'

Marcel Heller invites Mr Fresco into his consultation room. His partner man-
oeuvres the wheelchair through the door. Mr Fresco is slumped forward. 'Good
morning Mr Fresco. How are you feeling today,' Dr Heller asks, trying to establish contact. Mr Fresco does not respond. His partner says that things are
difficult. Mr Fresco had fallen out of bed this morning. Usually he sleeps all day
and then prowls round the house at night. She is worried that he will fall down
the cellar stairs. Last week he went down to the cellar to defecate. Yesterday
he urinated on the windowsill. Taking care of him is a full-time job. She asks
about the latest X-rays and the doctor tells her that his condition is deteriorating
rapidly. She says that she took him to a show on Tuesday and that he was
completely normal there, friendly to everyone, making jokes. If the doctors had
seen him there they would not have recognized him, she says. She wants to
know why they cannot give him more chemotherapy.

Dr Heller phones Sanne Wolfensperger to arrange for home care. He has to
persuade the partner to accept. They have a right to six weeks' home care

assistance and she wants to 'save this for the final weeks'. Dr Heller tells her that these *are* the final weeks. She cries. She knew he would die, but not *that* soon. She had been thinking in terms of years rather than weeks.

'Do we have to come back to the hospital?' she asks.

'Your GP can do everything that we can do in this phase,' Dr Heller says.

'I don't think so,' she says. He only looks at the outside; you can look inside as well. He doesn't have X-rays and chemotherapy.'

'We'll phone him and tell him what the situation is,' Dr Heller says. 'He's still one of our patients, so he's always welcome in the hospital. But the GP can do everything that is necessary.'

'Nurse,' Mr Fresco croaks, opening his eyes and looking at me. 'Are you free later?'

The attraction of the hospital for patients for whom treatment options have been exhausted

At the end of Part III I described how patients for whom all treatment options in the hospital have been exhausted are transferred back to their GP. At this stage in the illness doctors inform patients that there is nothing more they can do for them and that whatever is left to be done can be carried out just as efficiently by the GP. The assumption is that home – in a familiar environment and surrounded by loved ones – is the best place to die. Hospital specialists usually tell their patients at this time that they do not have long to live. 'That means that you don't have much time left,' is how they usually phrased it. The approaching death of a patient was not always made this explicit, however. But they did always say that if there were things that needed arranging, now was the time to take action.

I was struck by the fact that in this phase many patients and their families had difficulty in breaking their connection with the hospital. They had become used to – and even attached to – the routine of hospital visits. The doctors were familiar, and it was not exceptional that by the time they reached the final stage of their illness, patients had a more intimate relationship with the hospital specialist than with their GP. Part of the reason for this is that during the long treatment they had much more contact with the specialist than with their GP. Later, when they were sent home to die, it was difficult to re-establish the relationship with the GP.

Leaving the hospital also means an end to patients' interaction with the nurses, with whom both they and their relatives have often developed relationships. For most patients and their partners this is their first confrontation with a serious illness and everything is new and unknown and this is frightening and threatening. The nurses have experienced patients through good times and bad times and as a result a certain intimacy and trust has developed. But the nurses also provide practical advice. In Chapter 2 the nurse Mark van Rossum remarks that patients' partners have a lot of worries of their own. They have an acute need for information about what is going to happen, about whether new symptoms are related to the disease. Mrs Wessels thought it was wonderful to open her heart to the nurses and to discuss the problems involved in caring for her husband. Nurses are the ideal conversation partners: they are expert, understanding and accessible.

Leaving the hospital also means severing contact with fellow patients. There were periods in which groups of patients met each other every week and kept each other company in the waiting room. I have already described how these relationships can be both supportive and confrontational. Many patients and – perhaps especially – their partners felt a need to meet and discuss with others in the same situation. There were exceptions, of course, but for these reasons many patients and their partners found leaving the hospital difficult.

Finally, breaking contact with the hospital was also a symbolic separation, a separation from the idea of possible cure.

Contrasts and tensions between GPs and hospital specialists

During the illness trajectory the distance between patient and GP increases. This is not only a question of 'losing touch'. Tensions often developed in the relationship between GP and patient. Patients and their relatives frequently thought that the GP had underestimated the symptoms and referred them to the hospital too late. They felt that if the GP had acted earlier then the cancer would not yet have spread and might still have been curable. Sometimes patients and their relatives said that after the diagnosis they had heard nothing more from the GP, which either made them disappointed or angry. Mr and Mrs Dekker already mentioned this in Chapter 1.

Another complaint was that the GP had told them what was wrong in words that were too harsh. I often had the impression that GPs were more open about the prognosis than hospital specialists, but patients and their relatives did not always value this. The partner of one patient had told the GP that they were planning to go to Lourdes. The GP had advised them to go immediately otherwise it would be too late. The partner complained bitterly about what she saw as the GP's tactless and insensitive approach.

Part of the problem is that GPs are often the first stop in a long series of consultations with different doctors and there is a tendency to cast them in the role of scapegoat and blame them for all the subsequent suffering. The hospital specialist, on the other hand, is cast in the role of hero. He was never blamed for a late diagnosis. On the contrary, he was seen as doing everything possible to limit the damage. The specialists offered solutions; they could *do* something about the illness.

The demonization of the GP developed further in the hospital. I often heard patients and their relatives complain that the specialist had told them a completely different story from the GP. The GP had usually given the impression that there was no hope, whereas the specialist had said that there was hope. Various patients in my study told me that their GP disagreed with chemotherapy, particularly in the context of clinical trials. Sometimes GPs advised their patients to decline such therapy. When these patients decided to accept therapy anyway and the results turned out to be positive, this vindicated their decision and increased their trust in the hospital. It was striking that patients often described these successes as resulting from the personal efforts of a particular specialist. Patients often said things like, 'If you only knew how much Dr Liem has done for me,' or 'Dr Veerman has worked so hard; he's cured me.'

The GP pales next to the specialist's technical know-how. 'GPs don't know a thing about modern techniques,' patients often complained. The specialists tended not to contradict these ideas, and indeed they sometimes even initiated them. GPs and specialists also have different interests. Not only do specialists believe that the therapy they prescribe is useful, they also have a scientific interest: they need patients to carry out their trials.

The case of Mr Fresco illustrates that the high expectations that patients and their relatives cherish are part of the reason for the attractiveness of the hospital. Right up to the very end of life, patients and their relatives maintain their trust in the hospital's medical technology, a trust that sometimes becomes an obsession. The doctors told Mr Fresco and his relatives clearly that there were no other treatment options and that he did not have long to live. In spite of this his partner continued to bring Mr Fresco, who by now was more dead than alive, to the hospital, source of impressive scans and X-rays and chemotherapy. This is the power of medical technology, which supports patients' impression that specialists are 'real' doctors whose words are closer to the truth than those of 'mere' GPs.

Specialists are aware of the role of the hospital in the final phase of the illness trajectory. They advise patients, for whom all treatment options have been exhausted, to go back to their GP, but they also leave open the option of continuing to come to the hospital, which many patients do. Mr Wessels and his wife, for example, experienced these regular visits to the hospital – the trip in the ambulance, the long wait – as a day out. And Dr Liem allowed Mrs Wessels to phone him regularly.

Mr Fresco's GP

I look at my watch. It is quarter past five. The door swings open and Dr van Zomeren strides through the waiting room. 'Ms The,' he says giving me a firm handshake. 'Let's go into my office.' I follow him into a room full of books and papers. He takes a seat behind a large desk. With my tape recorder on the desk between us he tells me about his patient. It turns out that Dr van Zomeren was originally the GP of Mr Fresco's younger brother, Giovanni. One day Giovanni had asked Dr van Zomeren if he could help his brother, Carlos, who had been abandoned by his own GP.

'I didn't know he was terminal,' Dr van Zomeren says. 'I didn't know anything about his lung cancer. The first time I saw him was a few months ago. He phoned and asked if I could come and see him because he was coughing up blood. I went to see him and heard the whole story. He'd had a couple of courses of chemotherapy, everything was great and he had all kinds of plans. I listened to his lungs and whole sections were not functioning. He was terminal. I'd received some information from the previous GP, but not much. That's how it goes. As soon as patients find themselves in the grip of an academic hospital then you lose sight of them. The hospital specialists take over the check-ups and the GP no longer has a role. I only became involved when the hospital abandoned Carlos Fresco . . .' Dr van Zomeren falls silent as he reads Mr Fresco's file. 'Yes,' he continues, 'it was when it became clear that the chemotherapy wasn't working.'

'Progression under chemotherapy,' I mumble.

'Yes, that's what they call it. One evening Carlos was referred to the hospital by the GP on duty. I went to see him in the hospital. I decided to talk to the ward doctor, to introduce myself and to find out what they were planning to do with him. It wouldn't be the first time that they told a patient in that condition that the GP might be prepared to carry out euthanasia.' Dr van Zomeren laughs loudly. 'That was a very different case, but also from the Ruysdael Clinic. Yes, I had a very serious chat with them about that one. These days I want to know exactly what the situation is. I don't want to be a mere extension of the specialists.

'So I wanted to check with the ward doctor what they had found, what medication they were giving and whether there was indeed nothing more they could do for him. I thought they should send him home as soon as possible. I explained to the specialist that I thought that it was much more pleasant to die at home. People are conceived at home, they're born at home and I think they should be able to die at home. So he was discharged.

'Carlos Fresco had a girlfriend. They'd been together for ten, 15 years, and Carlos had promised her various things. Very complicated. He'd been spending money; things were not as they should be financially. Brother and sister Fresco and the girlfriend were as wary of each other as cats stalking the same prey. I tried to get him to see a solicitor but that didn't work out, so the real problems are still to come. You could say that at the moment there's an armed truce.

'I did manage to let him die peacefully. I increased the morphine slightly and things went very quickly.'

'How often do you visit terminal patients like Mr Fresco?' I ask.

Dr van Zomeren looks at Mr Fresco's file. 'I went to see him on the 2nd of February, then again on the 8th, the 12th, the 18th, 19th, 22nd, 23rd . . .'

'That's the day he came to the out patient clinic?'

'Why do they have to drag someone who's almost dead to the outpatient clinic?' Dr van Zomeren says, sighing. 'If they'd have asked me I'd have advised against it, but that girlfriend clutched at every straw. In cases like that those guys in the hospital should be much clearer that there's no chance of a cure.'

'The doctors in the hospital did say that but . . .'

'But it didn't get through to them, did it? I know, it just didn't penetrate.'

'Mr Fresco's partner asked whether they should come back again,' I say. 'The doctors said that it wasn't necessary but that they were always welcome if they felt the need.'

'Exactly,' Dr van Zomeren says. 'Friendly, very friendly, always welcome. But by saying that you deprive them of a good death. They remain focused on medical solutions, and that's why I'm opposed. You don't give them a chance to organize the things they need to organize. But I admit it's difficult. I recently told my own father this and he had difficulty coping. He's a retired GP, almost 90. At Christmas he asked me to feel his liver. It was grossly enlarged. I said, "Doesn't look too good, does it? Primary tumour or metastases. In either case it's the end". He couldn't take it. He'd seen whole villages of people die but he couldn't take it. I had to cover things up a bit. Shortly after that I told him that his liver was bigger still. A week later he was dead. Carlos knew how bad it was. He was putting on a brave face for his girlfriend.'

'He once said that if he had a gun he'd put an end to it. Did he ever mention that to you?' I ask.

'He never requested euthanasia, if that's what you mean. And if he had requested it, it wouldn't have been necessary. In his condition, a slight pneumonia and you're gone. I wouldn't have given him antibiotics if he'd developed a fever.

'I personally think that cytostatic drugs are a very dubious therapy. It wrecks you. When patients come to me, diagnosed with cancer, metastases, and ask me what to do I tell them – and this is revolutionary, but I don't mind getting into a debate with the professors – they can either let themselves be wrecked by cytostatic drugs in a year or die safely in a year of two [sic], with only a small chance that the cytostatic drugs will save them. I still have to see the first patient with metastases who has received cytostatic drugs and has a five-year survival. I've been a GP for 25 years and haven't seen one yet.'

'Earlier you said that once patients fall into the clutches of the hospital you hardly see them again.'

'Yes, that's correct. Listen, Carlos Fresco had lung cancer. In cases like that the first question is whether you can operate. That's only possible in a small number of cases, and if it's not a possibility then you have to make sure you guide the patient to a not too painful end. One of the problems in lung cancer is when the tumour eats into nerves in the chest. That's very painful. It's useful to give patients like that something to make the cancer less aggressive. Cytostatic drugs are useful in those cases. But it doesn't have a therapeutic effect; it won't give them another ten years of life. And in other cases it's just to be able to say that your patient lived a few months longer than someone else's did. It's statistics. It's not humane. In such cases you have to do things in consultation with the patient.'

'How?' I ask.

'You say to them, "Okay, you've got throat cancer, but you've got things to organize, your will, the grandchildren have to come over from Australia. That's important. We'll give you a feeding tube, so you have the chance to do all that. But you can remove it yourself if you want to. No one will complain. It means you'll soon die of hunger and dehydration. After a couple of days you won't feel the hunger any more. Thirst is nasty, but you can alleviate it by sucking ice cubes. You'll weaken and you'll die." That's what you tell them. You have to give them that freedom.' He looks at me fiercely.

'And in Carlos Fresco,' he continues, 'you just saw that dreadful survival obsession: if only I can find the right cytostatic drugs then I'll be saved. Rubbish! I try to emancipate my patients. I prepare them for the discussions they're going to have in the hospital. I tell them they're going to miss half of what's said. I tell them to have a list of questions ready, to insist on answers. I advise them to think rationally. And I try to show them that life is a game. Listen, Carlos Fresco had smoked 60 cigarettes a day all his life. And it's not as though no one knows that that carries certain risks. You have to look at it honestly: you played the game and you lost. In that way you prevent them ending up on diet therapy, or consulting a homeopath or drinking Norwegian alder tea. If they really want to that's okay with me, but I want them to be realistic.

'I don't have much in Carlos's file, but I could talk about him all day. That's the nice thing about my profession. I know things about him that a specialist would never learn. They don't know the patients in their everyday surroundings. How did they meet Carlos? As a case of metastasized lung cancer. That's all. If a specialist knows more about a patient than that then it's pure coincidence. Hopeless! I see things differently, that's why I became a GP. I see a patient and wonder what's wrong with him and whether I can help. That's what I like about my job. But it's frustrating when your efforts to help are blocked, and that happens often in practice.'

'You mean by the doctors in the hospital?' I ask.

'Yes, among others. But also by the patients themselves. The counselling isn't fair either. GPs should be present at the first discussion in the hospital about the treatment options. Patients look up to the specialist; they don't ask the right questions. They avoid the real issues. The specialists will never say, "You're going to die, that's one thing you can be sure of". They give the impression that if you come and let them treat you then . . .' Dr van Zomeren's voice trails off.

The GP's frustration

Reading through my data I realized that during my study of the illness trajectory of small-cell lung cancer the GP had been largely invisible. GPs play a central role in the initial phase of the illness, before diagnosis, but then the hospital specialists take over and the GP disappears from view. Some GPs still see their patients regularly, but for most contact is limited. The specialists informed GPs in writing about treatment and they telephoned in the case of important developments such as a recurrence or when the patient had reached the final stage of the illness.

My only information about the attitudes and behaviour of GPs came from the patients, their relatives and the hospital doctors. I almost never encountered them myself in the hospital. Dr van Zomeren, Mr Fresco's GP, was the first GP I encountered in the hospital. I later met him again at Mr Fresco's home. On both occasions we had a short conversation and he expressed interest in my work. I made an appointment with him because I wanted to hear the GP's perspective and make GPs more visible in my narrative.

Dr van Zomeren is critical of the hospital's approach, but he is not as idiosyncratic as he might seem. His views seemed to fit into the general line of criticism I had already heard attributed to other GPs. Moreover, I later interviewed four other GPs and they all had similar views. For their part, the specialists were also critical of GPs. This related mostly to the latter's medical-technical competence. The most common complaint was that GPs were not knowledgeable about modern chemotherapy; that their criticism applied to chemotherapy that was long obsolete. Not recognizing recurrence, and in particular brain metastases, was another criticism.

Usually GPs have known patients longer and know their families and social situations better than specialists. Dr van Zomeren first met Mr Fresco a year after the hospital specialists and yet he knew more about him and his social context than they did. This difference is therefore not related to the duration of contact but to a difference in perspective. In Dr van Zomeren's narrative there is a clear tension between himself and the specialists. This is largely due to the fact that the GP has a different idea about what constitutes proper treatment during the final phase of life. Frank (1995: 83) explains the GP's feeling of powerlessness through the example of a friend. This GP was dissatisfied about the way one of his patients was dying of cancer. He did not have a problem with the fact that she was dying – everyone has to die sometime and many die, like this patient, while still young. What he did find difficult, was having to watch while his patient was absorbed into the world of the hospital specialists who refused to accept that she was dying and continued to carry out tests. Frank's GP complains that, in addition to being a waste of resources, this approach did not help the patient to find her way towards a good death. There is no room for other narratives because Medicine's hope displaces these. This is exactly what so frustrated Dr van Zomeren. Patients like Mr Fresco do not have the opportunity to take any other course than that of treatment and hope prescribed by the hospital.

Dr van Zomeren tries to emancipate patients, as he puts it. He prepares them for what is to come and emphasizes that they should be realistic in their expectations regarding treatment and outcomes. Often this does not help and the doctor loses his patients to the hospital. Patients want to believe in wonders and they devote themselves to therapy. What the hospital promises is better than what GPs have to offer. Given their completely different idea about how this phase of the illness should be managed, it is often difficult for GPs to see their patients being carried along from one therapeutic solution to another on a wave of optimism. It is even more difficult when, in the very final phase, the hospital returns the dying patient to the care of the GP. It is also difficult for patients and their relatives to have to return to the GP who was so critical about therapy with the knowledge that he was probably right after all.

Of course, this by no means applies to all GPs and patients, and I have sketched the contrasts rather sharply. However, in many cases these mechanisms were at work to a greater or lesser extent.

12 Parting

Mr Dekker's parting

[17 December] Late in the afternoon I hear from Mark van Rossum that Mr Dekker has been brought to the hospital in an ambulance. He is accompanied by Vera and Johan. When he sees me he weeps and takes my face in his callused hands.

'It's finished, it's all over, it's the end. I can't go on any more,' he cries. 'I thought I'd never see you again. I told the children to go and look for you.'

'I knew that you were coming. And you know I always look you up when you are in the hospital,' I say, trying to calm him.

'I wasn't sure I'd be able to make it to the hospital,' he says. 'I can't fight it any more. I'm in terrible pain. It keeps me awake at night. They have to give me something for the pain. I've got a special bed downstairs at home because I can't get up the stairs any more. Rietje sleeps with me in the living room.' I take his hand. 'We all know I'm not going to get better,' he continues. Rietje and I have arranged everything. We've bought graves and I've told her exactly how I want the memorial service.' Vera takes his other hand. 'I don't think the last course of treatment has helped much. I came to the hospital to find out how my blood is.'

Dr Heller arrives with Mr Dekker's file under his arm. 'How are things?' he asks.

'Not good,' Mr Dekker says.

'What exactly is not good?' Dr Heller asks.

'Everything.'

Dr Heller nods. 'We'll have to decide what to do about the treatment,' he says. 'At the moment we can't give you any chemotherapy because your blood's not good.'

'I have the impression that the therapy worked at first,' Mr Dekker says. 'But the pain has returned. Also in my head. Can you please give me something for the pain, doctor?'

'We don't think he needs the chemotherapy anymore,' says Vera in a clear, sober voice. 'Not just to drag things out a bit longer, and especially not when he's in pain.'

'I want to delay that decision until after Christmas,' Dr Heller says. 'Maybe his blood will have recovered by then. In the meantime you can think things over. I also want to make an X-ray, at least if you agree. I'll leave that up to you.'

'Rather not,' Mr Dekker says. 'If I have to, okay, but preferably not.'

Dr Heller nods. 'I'll prescribe morphine for the pain. Then you can phone after Christmas for a new appointment.'

'My wife will call,' Mr Dekker says. 'I'm surprised you can do this job,' he says to me once Dr Heller has left and we are waiting for the ambulance to take him home. 'Isn't it terribly difficult having to associate with patients day-in and day-out?'

'Sometimes,' I say. 'But usually I enjoy it.'

He shakes his head. 'I wouldn't manage,' he says. 'I'm not sure I'll be coming back to the hospital,' he continues carefully.

'Shall I come and see you at home?' I suggest.

'Would you?'

'Yes, if you're not coming here anymore. But only if it's okay, because I hear you have a lot of visitors.'

'If you come I'll throw them all out. When are you coming?'

'Shall I phone your wife and make an appointment?' I say.

'Fine,' he says. When the ambulance arrives he strokes my hand. 'You've always been good to me,' he says.

[20 December] When I phone to make an appointment Vera answers. 'My uncle died early this morning,' she says. I suddenly realize what he was trying to tell me the last time I saw him in the hospital. Now I will never be able to tell him what all our meetings and discussions meant for me. The thought makes me sad. Mrs Dekker invites me round the next day. When I arrive the atmosphere is familiar, almost pleasantly cosy. We discuss the events of the past year; Mrs Dekker shows me photos. I stand with her in front of the coffin in the living room and say goodbye to Mr Dekker. This time consciously.

Consciously taking leave

Mr Dekker knew that he was going to die and accepted this.[1] And he took leave consciously.[2] This happened in various ways. From an early stage he

1 Kübler-Ross (1969) claims that almost all patients know when they are dying, whether they have been informed or not. Kellehear (1992: 80) argues that awareness of death is desirable and important as a basis for the four elements of what he calls 'good death'.
2 This does not necessarily mean that he accepted death (Kellehear 1992: 74).

was worried about what would happen to his wife and step-children after his death. He discussed this with Vera and Johan and they promised to help their step-mother. He also asked his sister to help. He and his wife saw a solicitor to sort out legal matters. He bought a plot in the cemetery and discussed funeral arrangements. The family talked a lot about the past; they looked at photo albums and relived good and bad times together.

The accident that left Mrs Dekker disabled and deprived Johan and Vera of their mother cast a shadow over the family. After their parents had separated Vera and Johan had not seen their real father again. In the final phase of his life Mr Dekker felt that because the children were losing him he should make an effort to renew their contact with their real father and heal the rift. He phoned their father in Germany and invited him to come to their home. The two men had a long discussion, no one quite knew what about. The meeting between Johan, Vera and their father was strained, but it was important for them that Mr Dekker gave his blessing and expressed the hope that they make an attempt to heal the rift.

Mr Dekker also said goodbye to me, even though I was not aware of this at the time. He had become someone I cherished. Although death and dying were central in my study, I had not wanted to admit to myself that he was dying, even though I really knew all along. I had not experienced this before; Mr Dekker was the first of 'my' patients to die. In the case of Mr Wiersema I saw this much more clearly, even though he had become equally dear to me, and I had the chance to say goodbye.

The death of a fellow patient

[12 January] 'Mr Wiersema is in room 101,' the nurse Lotte Kremer informs me. 'He's been admitted for a blood transfusion.' When I enter the room I am shocked by his thin, pale face framed by the pillows. Next to the bed are two medical students trying to insert an infusion needle. On the other side stands the nurse responsible for his care. The ward doctor, with more medical students and nurses in his wake, is doing rounds. They have stopped at the bed opposite Mr Wiersema's. It hurts to see him like that, exposed to what at that moment I experience as medical violence. I know his fear and loathing of the hospital, especially of being admitted on the ward. I want to leave and come back later when it is quieter, but he looks up and sees me. His greeting is hearty. 'Hey, Anne-Mei,' he says, immediately followed by, 'Dekker has gone'.

'I know,' I say.

'I saw him on the Friday,' Mr Wiersema talks through the din of all the medical activity around him. He holds his head inclined so that he can see me between the medical students. 'He told me it was finished,' he continues, tears in his eyes. 'I couldn't attend the funeral, and that really bothers me. I was too sick; I had terrible fever. We phoned though.'

The student moves Mr Wiersema's arm. 'It's difficult to get the needle in,' he says. The doctor is finished with the other patient and the procession comes toward Mr Wiersema's bed.

'I'll see you later,' I say, and slip out of the room.

I return an hour later with a medical student who has to take an illness history. The student sits next to the bed. Mr Wiersema looks at me and pats the bed next to him. 'Come and sit a bit closer,' he says. He talks about the past few weeks; a stream of words flows. He has hardly eaten; no appetite. That is why he has lost so much weight. He did not complete the radiotherapy because he was too ill and too weak. A few days ago he wiped all his pills off the table and onto the floor. There were so many he no longer knew which pills were for what. He had had enough and stopped taking them. 'I'm devastated by Dekker's death,' he keeps repeating, sadly. In between the student asks his questions: When did you fall ill? What were the symptoms? They sound trite. 'Do I have to answer all these questions?' Mr Wiersema says, slightly irritated. The student apologizes; those are the rules. I ask whether I should come back later, but he shakes his head.

He talks about his work. He is still on sick leave. The firm does not want to lose him. He is supposed to train a batch of new recruits in March. He thinks he might not be able to manage that. He has to get better first, then he will definitely be back at work. 'You can be sure of that,' he says confidently. He talks about how strong he was before the illness, how he lived for his work. He was always busy, hated being inactive, hated his bed. He always had a good appetite, ate mountains of potatoes smothered in gravy.

When the medical student has left he talks about the past few weeks. His voice trembles as he tells me how he could hardly cope. His eyes dart about the room as he repeats, 'What can I do? What can I do?' But he still has hope; he still wants to fight. There is no room for discussion about his actual prospects. He knows and is scared, but does not want to talk about it.

Resuscitation

[13 January] When I go to see Mr Wiersema the next morning the door of his room is closed. There has been a failed resuscitation attempt, I hear someone say. 'Who is it?' I keep asking the nurses running back and forth along the corridor. No one answers. Mr Wiersema is not in his room so I go looking for him. I eventually find him, scared and swearing in his bed, between the large plants in the day room. Relieved, I almost throw my arms around him. He has decided he must go home today, with or without the doctor's blessing. 'You're supposed to get better in hospital,' he says, 'but I'm only getting worse. It turns out that it was a patient sharing Mr Wiersema's room who had had a cardiac arrest.

[Rounds] 'Joop Wiersema, born in '41,' Dr Bolhuis begins. 'COPD, allergy. February last year diagnosed with a small-cell lung carcinoma in the left upper lobe, metastases in the mediastinum and liver. Extensive disease. He's had six courses of cisplatinum and etoposide in the context of a trial. Brain metastases in November. Patient broke off radiotherapy. Has had fever and has now been admitted for a blood transfusion. We are going to discharge him when the fever subsides. He has stopped taking his medication.'

'Why is he so rebellious?' asks Maarten Rutgers, junior doctor on the lung ward. 'Is he angry or distressed?'

'He's not happy that different doctors keep telling him different things,' Dr Bolhuis says.

'He's angry,' Dr Rutgers concludes. 'He knows he's going to die and that can cause depression. That's why he's taking it out on those around him.'

'Mr Dekker died,' Lotte Kramer, the nurse, says. 'They always shared a room. It's the first thing he talked about when he was admitted.'

'That's understandable,' Dr Rutgers says.

'Shouldn't we discuss a DNR order in the case of this patient?' Lotte Kramer asks.

'That's difficult,' Dr Rutgers says.

'But if something happens we need to know what we're supposed to do,' Lotte Kramer insists.

'I understand. In theory I think that a DNR order is appropriate in the case of a small-cell lung carcinoma with brain metastases. What do you think, Diederik?' He looks at the supervisor.

'Yes,' Dr Bron says, nodding. 'It sounds plausible.'

'But if you put that decision in writing then you're supposed to discuss it with the patient,' Dr Rutgers says. 'It could have an effect on the patient. In the current situation it could be traumatic.'

'The chance that he will have a cardiac arrest is very small,' Dr Bron says.

'Patients often interpret a decision like that as meaning that we're going to do nothing more for them,' Dr Rutgers says. 'You can discuss a decision like that with some patients but not with others.'

'Perhaps this patient still hopes that . . . you know,' Dr Bron says, shrugging. 'And then we'd be taking away his last hope.'

'The question is whether you should discuss this kind of decision with the patient at all,' says Dr Cardozo. 'It's a medical decision taken on medical grounds. After all, what do you do when you're called in the night because a patient with a small-cell lung carcinoma with brain metastases is having a cardiac arrest? You don't hurry.'

'Marcel Heller, Ronald Veerman and Guido Liem have a different view,' says Dr Rutgers. 'They think that as long as the patient's being treated you have to resuscitate.'

'A DNR order would affect other things as well,' Dr Cardozo says.

'That's a point. It's often said that if we're not going to resuscitate then we shouldn't treat either, though they are two different things. And that's difficult to sell to the patient. Imagine saying, "We're doing everything we can, except if you have a heart attack, in which case we won't do anything." I don't know how we can sell a decision like that.'

That afternoon Mr Wiersema informs Dr Rutgers that he assumes he will be discharged later the same day. Dr Rutgers agrees reluctantly.

Anger and resistance

Mr Wiersema's final weeks were quite different from those of Mr Dekker. He and his wife did not speak of solicitors and there was no leave-taking. Although Mr Wiersema's condition deteriorated rapidly he never spoke of his approaching death. Indeed, the subject of death was taboo. He talked about persevering and not giving up hope. He became grim and, just like Mr de Jager in Chapter 10, increasingly unrealistic. He had always repeated the narrative of hope in its many variations: 'You just wait and see, next year I'll be back at work,' and 'This summer I'll be on my boat'. What else could he say? He would not be able to cope otherwise.

Some change was visible, however. He was sad and scared, and he expressed this through increasing resistance to both the hospital policy and his GP. He refused radiotherapy and stopped taking his medication. The deaths of Mr Dekker and a fellow-patient sharing the same room had upset him. The death of Mr Dekker was particularly hard to deal with. Not only did it deprive him of a friend, it also confronted him directly with death and served to remind him of his own approaching death. He was constantly reminded of this in the hospital, where Mr Dekker's death had left an atmosphere of sadness and loss among many of the patients who had known him. The unexpressed thought of many was: who will be next? From the discussion before rounds it was apparent that if it had been Mr Wiersema and not the other patient who had had a cardiac arrest then he would not have been resuscitated. This fact, even though Mr Wiersema was not aware of it, tended to make his fears more real.

The pre-rounds discussion about resuscitation and how this should be presented to the patient was typical. As a result of a failed resuscitation attempt, general resuscitation policy was discussed more intensively than usual, and this lead on to further discussion about the desirability of dashing patients' hope. Various views were aired, but no decision was reached on what should be done.

Mr Dekker's shadow

[26 January] Dressed and sitting on a chair in the waiting room, Mr Wiersema looks better and less vulnerable than the last time I saw him in bed on the ward. When he is called into the infusion room, Mrs Wiersema stays behind with me.

She tells me that they still cherish hope that the treatment will work, even though they now talk of 'extending life' rather than 'cure'. She says she now understands what they mean in obituaries when they say that someone had died 'after a long struggle'. She says he becomes really angry when people say he should fight against the illness. What do they think he is already doing?

Mrs Wiersema has spoken to Mrs Dekker. She experienced the meeting as confrontational. Mrs Dekker gave well-meaning advice. 'I think you should have the coffin at home before the funeral, it's so much nicer,' Mrs Dekker had said. Mrs Wiersema tells me that Joop hates the hospital. The resuscitation had been very unpleasant and he hadn't had a moment's peace, what with all the medical students constantly bothering him. But Dr Liem had asked him, and he couldn't refuse a request from Dr Liem. After all, Dr Liem allows him to call at any time if there is a problem.

Mr Wiersema spends most of the day in bed. He is still losing weight, even though the last set of X-rays looked reasonable. Dr Liem said that he was getting more air. That was good news for Joop. When he came home from the hospital he said he could do with a nice pork chop. He hadn't eaten one for weeks.

Later Sandra Koster tells me that her father and Mr Wiersema embraced each other when they met in the X-ray Department. This was their first encounter since Mr Dekker's death. 'Now we've only got each other,' they said. I had also noticed how they tried to cheer each other up, searching for reasons why things went wrong with Mr Dekker.

'Klaas Dekker was a special case,' Mr Wiersema said on one such occasion. 'Yes, he had a large tumour in his neck. It had spread everywhere,' Mr Koster agreed. Both men nodded wisely.

'Yes, when that happens you know you don't have long to go,' Mr Wiersema said.

But these discussions did not alleviate their worries. It had been a terrible shock that Mr Dekker, who had helped to pull everyone through with his indestructible humour and positive attitude, should be the first to succumb.

Sandra Koster tells me she has had a good discussion with Dr Liem. She now understands that her father is in 'the final phase'. At home things are difficult. Dr Liem said he was going to speak to her father as well. He explained that the chemotherapy was meant to improve Mr Koster's situation, but that it was up to him to decide whether it was worth it. 'I will be guided by what your father says,' Dr Liem said. Sandra is worried that it will come as a shock to her father to hear what the reality of the situation is. She says she will try and prepare him, but it is a huge responsibility.

'It's different to last time,' Mr Koster says later, as I sit next to him in the waiting room. 'Last time the doctor said, "the tumour has *gone*". Now he says, "the tumour is *stable*". That means it's still there. Strange thing is,' he continues after a long silence, 'he still keeps saying he's satisfied.'

'The funny thing is,' Dr Liem says to me a few minutes later, shaking his head, 'when patients are here they always pretend to be much better than when they are at home. Take Mr Koster for example. He always tells me he's feeling fine, not ill at all, not feeling nauseous, nothing. Then I hear from his daughter that he's a wreck, can hardly do anything. Why can't they just tell me that themselves?'

In a discussion with Dr Liem, Mr Koster says that he is having difficulty keeping up the chemotherapy. 'Why go on if it's not going to cure me? Nothing can stop this illness; it's a silent killer.' Mr Koster continues with chemotherapy nonetheless.

The silent killer and the address book

A few weeks later Mr Koster is admitted to hospital with a chemotherapy-induced 'dip'. His condition deteriorates rapidly. He spends most of the day in bed, in a dazed condition, wearing headphones. He listens to Ravel's Bolero continuously; his daughter has recorded it on both sides of the tape and the Walkman is auto-reverse. It is clear that Mr Koster is not going to survive much longer. The doctors do their best to get him into good enough shape to be discharged so that he can die at home. Then he has a lung haemorrhage. A nurse on the early morning shift finds him dead in bed, Ravel's Bolero still emanating loudly from the headphones.

On the day before the funeral I visit the Koster household to pay my respects. Mrs Bokjes accompanies me. Mr Bokjes had always shared a room with Mr Koster during first-line chemotherapy, but he refused to come along as the visit would be too confrontational. We sit around the table in the living room, a large flask of coffee between us. Sandra pours coffee, we help ourselves to sugar and milk. A packet of tobacco and cigarette papers are passed round. I look round the room. A wedding photo of Mr and Mrs Koster hangs on the wall. It does not hang straight and the white rectangle of wall behind it contrasts with the rest of the cigarette-smoke stained room. I feel ashamed and focus my attention back on the assembled group. Sandra's husband rolls a cigarette and passes the tobacco to her. After rolling one of her own she passes the packet to me. I shake my head.

'Great that you don't smoke,' she says. 'I wish I could stop.' I feel awkward. In the room on the opposite side of the corridor Mr Koster lies in his coffin, dead from lung cancer. We are all there to mourn his passing, and all except me are smoking. 'The silent killer,' I hear Mr Koster saying. I am painfully aware that by refusing to roll a cigarette, I have focused attention on smoking.

'I never really managed to start smoking,' I say, trying to sound casual, 'so I don't know about the difficulties in stopping.'

Sandra seems to feel the tension. 'They say that dad's cancer was caused by smoking,' she says. 'But I don't believe a word of it. Dad didn't believe it either. He worked hard all his life. *Really* hard. After mom died he sacrificed himself for us.' She sounds angry. 'There are so many other possible causes, like the chemicals they spray on plants.'

The argument is familiar. I remember Mr Wiersema slipping away from the ward for a surreptitious smoke, his half-smoked cigarette butt hidden in a matchbox. 'Do the doctors allow you to smoke?' I asked him. 'No, they say it's bad for you. They say it causes cancer, but I don't believe it. I've always worked hard; I did the work of three people. That's what caused it.' I also remember one of my discussions with Mr Dekker in the outpatient waiting room. He had been quiet for a while, but I had learnt that these silences were followed by discussion of a topic that was currently exercising him. He broke the silence by saying that he thought it unfair how smoking was being blamed for his illness. His own explanation was that it had been caused by air pollution and chemicals to which he had been exposed at work.

The strangest explanation, however, came from Mrs Fisher-Rijn, when I asked her why she thought she had got cancer. 'When I consulted the doctor about pain in my neck he tried to fix things,' she said. Something broke, I could hear it snap quite clearly.' She points to the exact spot on her neck.

'But what has that to do with lung cancer?' I asked.

'Well, it moved down into my lungs, of course,' she said impatiently, tracing the movement from neck to lungs with her hand.

'And then you got cancer?' I ask in disbelief.

'Precisely, that's how it got into my lungs.'

'When did that happen?'

'It must have been at least ten years ago. That's when I started coughing. Yes, I can tell you, I've carried it about with me for quite a while now.'

'Have you ever mentioned this to Dr Liem?'

'Yes. He doesn't believe me, though.' She straightens her skirt and looks me in the eye. 'But you can't expect him to, can you? He wasn't there at the time.'

The next morning I called by to pick up Mrs Bokjes on my way to Mr Koster's funeral. Mr Bokjes is just arriving home from the hospital in a taxi. I drink coffee with him in the garden while his wife is getting ready. 'Strange,' he says as he stares at a group of children cycling past. 'When we were all there on the ward together, I thought they were all stronger than me. But Dekker went, then Koster, and now Wiersema is not doing so well.' He removes a small address book from his pocket. 'Can you write your address in here?' he says, showing me a long list of names. 'For later, for her,' he whispers, gesturing toward where his wife is getting ready. 'So she knows where to send the cards, understand?' I nod.

'Do you think it'll go that fast?' I ask.

'That's precisely the question,' he says, shrugging. 'But I do want everything to be arranged when the time comes.'

Causal attribution and smoking

Patients tried to find reasons for their illness, particularly at the start, following diagnosis, and at the end, just before they died. It is at those moments that patients and their relatives tried hardest to answer the question: Why me? Relatives continued to be exercised by this question after the death of their loved one.

It is common knowledge that smoking is the main cause of lung cancer, but only very few patients admitted that smoking was the cause of their illness. It was difficult for them to admit, and difficult for their relatives to accept, that they themselves were responsible. Instead they explained the illness in terms of what I will call heroic self-sacrifice (working too hard, for example). Referring to Susan Sontag, Ten Kroode (1990) remarks that it is more difficult for cancer patients to admit their own responsibility for their illness than for the victims of a heart attack because cancer is considered to be a dishonourable disease.

However, the fact that patients refused to admit that smoking was the cause of their cancer did not mean that they were not aware of the connection. Mr Dekker was one of the many patients who stopped smoking immediately after diagnosis. Others continued to smoke but did so secretly. I never heard doctors attribute lung cancer explicitly to smoking. Dr Liem once told me that he thought it unnecessary to burden patients with feelings of guilt. Doctors only made the connection explicit when patients insisted. I also never heard doctors tell patients that they should stop smoking. This is not surprising, as it would not have made much difference.

Mr Wiersema does not show up at the outpatient clinic

[11 February] Mr Wiersema is on the outpatient appointment list but I do not see him in the waiting room. Suddenly I hear a sharp whistle. I turn round and see a slim woman with brown curly hair waving wildly. I do not recognize her and look around to see who she could be waving to. 'No,' she shouts, 'it's you. Don't you recognize me? Liesbeth Quint. You spent enough time at my bedside.' The recognition comes slowly. The last time I had seen her was months ago. She had been sick, weak and wasted, with a scarf hiding her bald head. There was no one at home to take care of her, so when she was discharged from hospital she had been admitted to a nursing home. When the cancer recurred soon after the completion of first-line chemotherapy she had told the hospital doctors and her GP that she no longer wanted to be treated; that she wanted euthanasia. After a number of discussions with Dr Heller she decided to try again. I had lost sight of her after that and, being familiar with the fate of most lung cancer patients, had assumed she was dead.

The contrast between the memory of the dying patient in the hospital bed and the healthy woman now standing opposite me is amazing. I have to restrain myself from blurting out, 'You're still alive!' Instead I stammer, 'I didn't recognize you.'

'I've been like this for almost a year now,' she says. 'The picture on the X-rays is stable.' She slaps her thigh and jokes that she is putting on so much weight that she has to go on a diet.

At lunchtime Dr Heller asks Dr Liem whether he has heard anything from Mr Wiersema. There was a rumour circulating in the waiting room that he was too ill to come to the hospital. 'Yes,' says Dr Liem nodding, 'His GP phoned yesterday to ask whether I had a problem with him taking over responsibility for Mr Wiersema. I said I thought it was a good idea.' When I talk to Dr Liem later he tells me that Mr Wiersema's condition has deteriorated rapidly and that he might die tonight.

'That's really fast compared to Mr Wessels,' I say.

'Yes, but that was a completely different case. Mr Wiersema had progression during treatment. In the case of Mr Wessels the therapy worked but he stopped because of the side effects. Mr Wessels reaped the benefits of therapy for a long time after he stopped.'

'But is there progression in Mr Wiersema?' I ask. 'I haven't heard anything about that.' I think back to the last discussions and Mr Wiersema celebrating with his pork chop.

'I haven't told them yet because the X-rays are still stable,' Dr Liem says. But during the years I have become sensitive to the subtle changes in the clinical picture of lung cancer. I think there is progression.'

In the coffee room the nurses Mark van Rossum and Titia de Bruin are chatting. Dr Heller has just poured a cup of coffee. He holds the pot up questioningly. 'You look a bit flushed,' he says.

'I saw Mrs Quint this morning, and I almost blurted out, "Are you still alive!"' I say. They all laugh. 'I wanted to find out what had happened,' I continue.

'That happens to us as well,' Titia de Bruin says. 'We're always discussing who's died and who hasn't. Sometimes we assume a patient is long dead and then suddenly they appear again.'

'I suddenly became painfully aware of the difference between how we talk among ourselves about these things and how we talk when the patient is present,' I say. 'We continually say to each other that a patient is not going to last much longer, but when the patient asks we refuse to be specific, never mind using the word death. You, Marcel, you wished Mr Wiersema a merry Christmas while telling me it would be his last. You didn't say *that* to Mr and Mrs Wiersema.'

'Yes, well,' Marcel says, 'that's just how things are.'

Mr Wiersema's parting

[13 February] Sunday morning the phone rings. 'Is that Anne-Mei?' a cracked voice asks. 'This is Hanneke Wiersema. It's the end; Joop is dying. Sorry to bother you in the weekend, but I thought you'd rather be told now than hear about it later.' All kinds of thoughts flash through my mind.

'Do you want me to call by?' I ask.

'Do you want to come?'

'I don't want to trouble you.'

'It's no trouble.'

'Then I'll come,' I say.

Later that day, when she opens the front door, Hanneke Wiersema takes my hand. 'Don't be shocked,' she says. 'You won't recognize him.' I try to prepare myself by thinking of the single rooms on the ward where I have seen other dying patients. I see their faces, smell their smell. I squeeze Mrs Wiersema's hand. We go into the room. Mr Wiersema is emaciated. She wakes him. 'Joop, it's Anne-Mei,' she says, raising her voice. 'Anne-Mei from the hospital.' He opens his eyes with difficulty. He looks at me and waves a hand weakly. 'I've come to say goodbye,' I say. 'We've shared such a lot. Your wife called and I'm happy about that.' He reaches out a hand and pulls me toward him with surprising strength, then he pushes me away. 'I'll leave you to rest,' I say. He is still the man I first met more than a year ago: fighting and denying. I am saddened by his lonely struggle.

Mrs Wiersema tells me that she now values the contact she has with Mrs Dekker. They are equal once again and can support one another. She has also been in contact with Mrs Bokjes, who had insisted that she also speak to Mr Bokjes. He had cried, saying, 'Oh Hanneke, I'll be next.' She regretted having talked to him, she says, because it had upset him. She remembers how confrontational contact with the Dekkers had been for her not so long ago.

She says that she and her husband had talked about the situation. She said that they had always found the doctors in the hospital honest. They had always been shown the X-rays and everything. Except the last time. Joop had asked for the X-rays but Dr Liem had simply said that he had already discussed them with Dr Meulman and that they were okay. The Wiersemas had been suspicious. They phoned the GP, who phoned Dr Liem, who told the GP that the X-rays looked okay but that he thought that things were nearing the end. The GP passed this information on to the Wiersemas.

'When Joop's condition suddenly deteriorated earlier this week I decided not to phone the hospital,' Mrs Wiersema continued. 'I knew they'd admit him, and he hates that. I decided to contact the GP and arrange things at home. And I must say, he's doing a fantastic job. He's phoned the hospital to let them know what's happening. We hadn't had much contact with our GP lately, and when we did he always gave us different advice to the hospital. That was unpleasant. But now he's a real support. He's prescribed morphine in case Joop is in pain. It's in the fridge, but fortunately he hasn't needed it yet. I've also been in touch with Natasha, the faith healer. She said Joop needed a flu vaccination. I didn't respond. I've always thought that he'd die when his time came, and that no one, either doctors or faith healers, would be able to do anything about it.

'The community nurse thinks I should tell Joop that he's dying. She says we should discuss it.' Over her shoulder I can look into the other room, where I see the end of the bed in which Mr Wiersema is dying. 'We've never discussed that,' she continues. Her hands tremble. 'He's never mentioned it. He's not the type to talk about things like that. Should I start discussing that *now*? Because he does know, you know. He's said a few times, "I want to be taken to The Woodlands." That's the cemetery near here, you know?'

[14 February] When I get home from work Mrs Wiersema calls to tell me that her husband died the previous evening. In his own way, he had said goodbye to his loved ones. 'I found a letter,' she says. 'A goodbye letter, telling me how he wants things to be organized, and what music he wants at the funeral. He also wrote what a good time he had had with me and the children, and that he wanted to thank us for everything. I found it between the insurance papers. He wrote it during the period that things started to deteriorate rapidly. I remember coming home one day to find him writing.'

Knowing and not knowing

To a large extent the illnesses of Mr Wiersema and Mr Dekker ran parallel: the shock of diagnosis, the commitment to treatment, the hope of cure, the disappointing and unexpected recurrence of the tumour. There were differences as well, though, especially in their experience of the illness. These became pronounced in the final phase. Earlier in this chapter I described these differences as they relate to the two main characters in this book: Mr Dekker who recognized and accepted approaching death, prepared himself, sorted out his affairs and said his goodbyes, and Mr Wiersema who never spoke of death, even to those closest to him.[3]

The fact that Mr Wiersema did not talk about death and claimed that he would be back at work when he recovered seem to suggest that he was not aware that he was dying. As I have discussed in Chapter 10, this is not necessarily the case. The awareness of dying can be latent and can vary depending on the context. Because of the complexity of psychological defence mechanisms, it is sometimes difficult to determine whether and to what extent an individual is aware (Kellehear 1992: 75).

I think that Mr Wiersema was well aware that he was dying. He could hardly not have been aware, given the nature and extent of his physical deterioration. But there are other signs. In spite of his increasing weakness he struggled to finish decorating the house, he wrote a goodbye letter to his wife, and on the 5th of December, when we met in the rain, he told me of his concerns for his wife and children after his death. Perhaps he never spoke of death because he wanted to protect them,

---

3 In Kellehear's study 54 per cent of the patients shared their awareness of dying with their partner (Kellehear 1992: 78).

perhaps he felt emotionally incapable of broaching such an emotional topic. Context is also important. When Mr Wiersema ran into me unexpectedly in the rain he was able to discuss death. Perhaps this was because I was an outsider who knew the situation. Maybe he felt that I was willing to listen.

So Mr Wiersema was aware that he was dying, so were his wife and children. But nobody spoke about it. And so, unlike Mr Dekker, he died alone.

Individual styles of living and dying

The difference between Mr Dekker and Mr Wiersema was not so much that the former was aware he was dying while the latter was not, but lay rather in the way in which they dealt with this awareness. The question here is why they dealt with the final phase of life so differently.

Part of the reason lies in differences in character and personality. Mr Dekker found it easier to accept the ups and downs of life; he was more adaptive. Some people seem to find it easier to adjust after disruptions in the normal routine of their lives; they do not experience them as personal insults. Perhaps this made it easier for Mr Dekker to accept that he was dying than for Mr Wiersema.

I was often struck by how the news of impending death could come as such a complete surprise, as though those involved had never considered the possibility. It was only the odd patient who was not surprised, like the religious patient who said that he had always considered life a temporary affair, a sort of apprenticeship from which he could be recalled at any time. He was not scared of death because it led to real life on the other side. It is difficult to say what the exact role of religion was in the patients I studied. Almost all of them were religious and scared of death. Mr Dekker was religious and accepted death; Mr Wiersema was also religious and did not.

The thought of death prompted different responses. Some patients looked back at their lives and were grateful, others emphasized the dark and negative aspects. Mr Wiersema worried about what the future had to offer, while Mr Dekker tried to live in the present and enjoy the time that remained, so that his family would have pleasant memories of the last weeks they spent together. Mr Dekker was used to confronting problems head-on; Mr Wiersema tended to avoid difficult situations. Mr Dekker could discuss emotions. The first time I met him on the ward he told me about his wife's accident and how he had experienced it. Mr Wiersema never mentioned emotional matters to me. Mrs Wiersema said that her husband had never been a talker, and he did not become one in the final stage of his life either.

Biography and development

In addition to personality and character, people's life experience – their biography – also play a role in how they cope. Mr Dekker recounted that after his wife's accident he came to realize that he was not invulnerable. Another patient told me that he had lost his fear of death after having worked for an undertaker. Earlier I described the few patients who had refused treatment. They had all been in contact with dying cancer patients through their work.

During this study I was struck by the extent to which particular experiences – and not only those before the illness – can alter people's attitudes. Take Mr Bokjes for example. He was a nervous individual and during first-line chemotherapy almost everything was just too much for him emotionally. However, shortly after the death of Mr Koster he was able to hold out his address book when his wife was not looking and ask me to add my address to the list of those to receive invitations to the funeral. I am sure that this boldness was a result of his experiences with fellow-patients. He had already seen several other patients passing along the same trajectory that he himself was following. He was aware of what was in store for him and was gradually getting used to the idea. I have already referred to this process of development, involving observation, experience and time.

Those close to the patient play an important role in this process. At the beginning of the book I described how Mrs Rogge's children did not allow her the chance to develop any hope of a cure. Each time she tried to focus too much on the doctor's optimistic words or apparently positive changes in the X-rays, her children reminded her of what had been said during the bad news interview. However, this is an exception and the opposite is usually the case. I have also described how patients and their relatives try to protect each other, and how they develop positive future scenarios together.

Mr Wiersema's funeral

[17 February] The auditorium of The Woodlands is full. Mr Wiersema's coffin is on the podium. I see Mrs Wiersema and her four children at the front. Joanne, the oldest daughter, looks round and sees me. She whispers something to her mother. Mrs Wiersema looks over her shoulder; I smile. She looks back sadly. A man in a grey suit takes his place behind the microphone. It is Mr Wiersema's boss from work. He talks of the hard worker, the devastating disease and, in particular, the sudden and unexpected end. After all, had he not constantly talked about returning to work?

Afterwards we move in a procession to the grave. I walk just behind the boss and a group of colleagues, picking up shreds of their conversation. 'That makes three who've died of cancer this year,' says the man on the boss's left. 'Yes,

Wiersema was the fourth,' says another. I find myself wondering who might be next.

When the coffin has been laid to rest and we have gone back inside, the undertaker asks us to let the family drink their coffee in peace before offering our formal condolences. After my coffee I cross over to Mrs Wiersema. She embraces me. 'How lovely that you've come,' she says. The children also embrace me and thank me. I wonder what for. I feel the urge to go outside. I need fresh air.

PART V

Conclusion

13 Conclusion and recommendations

Introduction

The unjustified optimism which patients with small-cell lung carcinoma cherished about recovery was the pretext for this study. Why were they optimistic in spite of knowing their situation was hopeless? And what was it in the communication between doctors, patients and nurses that caused patients to be oblivious to what was obvious to their care providers? In this chapter I summarize and comment on the answers to these questions. As I have done in the rest of the book, I let the conclusions follow the trajectory of my own discovery, characterized by its shift in perspective. I started out from an *informed consent perspective* and focused mainly on verbal communication, looking predominantly at what people said and how they said it. Following my own experience in the early stages of the study, I gave the reader the idea that 'there was something wrong with the communication,' and that the doctors were the guilty party. I then clarified the influence of the patient. As a result, it became clear why the communication and decision making processes happen as they do, and I introduced the *care perspective*.

Phases of the illness trajectory and the bad news interview

After having studied the illness trajectories of 30 patients with small-cell lung carcinoma in great detail, I know that not all patients are optimistic. In fact, patients are only optimistic during certain phases of their illness. The patients whose limitless optimism so surprised me at the beginning of my study, such as Mr van der Ploeg, with whom I opened this book, were in this optimistic phase. After the diagnosis of their illness, patients experience despair and go through an existential crisis. Optimism about the possibility of recovery develops during treatment and characterizes the remission phase of the illness in which the tumour recedes and the patient feels 'better'. When the tumour reappears or the patient's condition deteriorates, then this optimism gives way to despair. The alternating of optimism and despair is repeated during second-line chemotherapy, though the optimism now tends to be less extreme. During the course of the illness the patient's perception changes continually, as he gradually discovers that there are different phases in the development of his illness. This is partly due to the fact that his physical condition changes, but also because he learns more about the nature and course of his illness.

Another reason for patients' optimism is that they are not clearly informed about their prognosis. Doctors (and nurses) have this information but they generally keep it to themselves. Although patients visit the hospital frequently and regularly see the specialist, the total trajectory of the illness is seldom discussed. Only when it is medically necessary (i.e. immediately following diagnosis, when the tumour recurs and when nothing more can be done for the patient) does the doctor initiate a bad news interview and tell the patient about his long-term perspective.

During the first bad news interview (following diagnosis) the doctor informs the patient about the aggressive nature of the tumour and discusses the ultimately fatal outcome. He tells the patient that the chance of recovery is very slim. The communication in this first bad news interview has a number of striking characteristics. First, the specialist hardly dwells on the dynamic development that characterizes small-cell lung carcinoma, or the ways in which patients are likely to interpret this. During treatment the tumour 'disappears' from the X-rays and the patient interprets this as cure. The doctor does not warn the patient not to be unduly optimistic about this development, and does not mention that the tumour generally returns (repeatedly) after a short period of remission. At most he mentions that the tumour 'tends' to return.

Second, the interview is characterized by a sudden change of course: a rapid transition from counselling about the disastrous diagnosis to discussion of treatment. During the second (and longest) phase of the interview, the various treatment options, the treatment plan, and explanations about various details of the treatment are central. The major part of the interview is devoted to treatment, and the emphasis is on this. In comparison, counselling about the fatal diagnosis and the general prognosis pales. Both doctor and patient gratefully shift their attention from diagnosis to 'what can be done about it' (Bensing 1991).

Third, the prognosis is not shared with the patient. True, the doctor does mention the disastrous outcome, but he gives no idea of the actual time involved. Even when patients enquire explicitly about this, doctors are extremely reluctant to say anything specific. The patient is told that it is difficult to say anything general about prognosis because this depends on so many factors, which differ from one patient to another. 'You never know exactly how a patient is going to react to therapy,' I often heard doctors say. This tendency to individualize prognosis is widespread and in the literature it is interpreted as giving the patient the hope that he will do better than his fellow patients (de Swaan 1985; Costain Schou 1993: 252). Moreover, if the doctor pins himself to a specific prognosis, this entails the bizarre 'risk' that the patient will 'outlive' it.

While the course of the illness *does* differ from one patient to another, more *could* be said about the prognosis, despite the impression that doctors give to their patients.[1] Doctors (and nurses) discuss the prognoses of individual patients and the general prognosis of small-cell lung carcinoma among themselves. They also discussed this with me. As Dr Heller said, referring to Mr Wiersema, 'This will be his last Christmas'. There appear to be other reasons for doctors' reluctance to discuss prognosis with the patient. These are related to what they think is best for the patient. Many specialists think that it is not good for the patient to live with the knowledge that he is shortly to die (see Wagener 1996). They have learnt, and they believe, that it is wrong to deprive the patient of hope.

Here it is important to consider to what extent the interests of the patient are really central in this reluctance to discuss prognosis. Perhaps it is not so much that it is better for the patient not to hear about his prognosis, but better for the doctor not to have to reveal it. This is especially the case when the patient is not expecting bad news. It is well known that doctors experience talking about death as a heavy burden (see Taylor 1984). Doctors are at risk of becoming 'infected' by the patient's feelings of helplessness and uncertainty because they do not have ready answers to questions of life and death (Gelauff and Manschot 1997: 202). The amount of time they have and their emotional resources influence how and how much doctors inform patients. I empathize with this fully, and it is not my intention to point an accusatory finger at doctors who are confronted with the task of informing patients that they are going to die. I simply want to examine the reasons behind doctors' behaviour.

---

1 The odd patient with a small-cell lung carcinoma might survive a few months or a year longer than expected, but should these exceptions determine the provision of information more generally? In discussions about patients I was often struck how doctors used these exceptions to legitimize their actions. The nurses also pointed this out to me. An intensive care nurse once said: 'Specialists say: "five years ago I had a patient with the same clinical picture. We'd given up, but then decided to treat him anyway. When we'd finished he was well enough to *walk* home." ' The much larger group of patients who do not respond that radically to treatment are much more central in the nurses' memory. Differences in levels of responsibility and different kinds of contact with the patient are part of the reason for this.

In the period between the bad news interviews, during treatment and remission phases, the specialists 'follow' their patients; they adjust to the way the patient experiences his illness. Doctors seldom if ever broach the topic of the general course of the illness and its fatal outcome. They answer patients' questions about the future, but remain reserved about the prognosis. For example, if a patient is optimistic and enthusiastically tells the doctor about his plans for the future, then the doctor generally goes along with this. The doctor neither contradicts nor supports what the patient is really saying, 'I'm going to get better, doctor, aren't I?' Doctors say that they do not think it good to confront patients with hard clinical reality at such moments. They argue that the moment will come soon enough when the patient's long-term prospects have to be discussed, i.e. when the tumour recurs.

The various bad news interviews proceed in phases. In the second interview the doctor no longer says that he probably cannot cure the patient, but that the patient will not get better. He progressively becomes more open about the general course of the illness, the merely palliative nature of the therapy, and the prognosis. The doctor's counselling becomes clearer and his tone more decided. At the same time, the patient's need for information seems to increase; he is emotionally in a better position to cope with clinical reality. He asks more specific questions, is less satisfied with generalizations and gives the doctor more room to elaborate. In answer to persistent questions about the prognosis, the specialist is prepared to reveal more about the illness. He might inform the patient that the survival rate at two years is 20 per cent, for example. At this point the specialist is still reluctant to be specific about the time frame for the individual patient. However, when nothing more can be done for the patient in the hospital and he is referred back to his GP, the specialist will give the patient an individual prognosis. He might say something like, 'you should think in terms of months, perhaps even weeks,' or 'if you have things to organize, then you'd better do so now'.[2]

To a certain extent, there is never one single moment in which the doctor informs the patient about the bad news. We talk of the bad news interview but in fact it is more a series of discussions. The patient is given the information in doses. At the beginning of the process the patient visits the specialist for the first time, referred by the GP because of persistent symptoms. When the tumour recurs the patient comes to the specialist with symptoms, or for a general check-up, during which the recurrence of the tumour is discovered. At these points the diagnosis is clear and the

---

2 What happens is exactly what GP van Zomeren wanted: that patients are informed a few weeks in advance that they are going to die.

specialist informs the patient of his concerns. However, he cannot yet say anything with certainty without further tests, such as scans or bronchoscopy, and the specialist who carries out the tests often gives the patient some inkling of the results.[3] The patient then goes back to the doctor to discuss the results. Sometimes the doctor informs the patient of the results by phone. In addition to these verbal preparations for the bad news interview, there are also various non-verbal signs, which point to what is to come. For example, the patient comes for tests, the next appointment is in the oncology department, then the doctor makes a special appointment to see the patient and his family to discuss the test results.

In the literature the bad news interview is described as a 'marathon session,' implying that the patient is told everything in a single go. I have shown that this is not the case with small-cell lung carcinoma; it seldom occurs that everything is revealed in a single session and the provision of the bad news is a gradual process. It is difficult to imagine that this is different in other hospital departments, in other hospitals or in the case of other types of cancer. Diagnostic tests always need to be carried out, and it seems likely that in the case of other, slower forms of cancer, the provision of information would be spread over an even longer time period.

By distancing myself from the term 'marathon session,' I do not wish to imply that the information content of the bad news interview is low; in fact it is possibly too high for patients, given their emotional state. People have difficulty coming to terms with the news that they are going to die soon, whether this is presented in a single session or spread over numerous sessions, and in this sense it is always a marathon session. Specialists utilize the natural course of events (symptoms, diagnostic tests, results) consciously as a counselling strategy. Through this process they prepare patients for the bad news, allowing them gradually to get used to the idea that they have cancer or a recurrence of a tumour. In fact, the patient is not usually told the bad news during the bad news interview, but rather the information that he has received earlier – through the concern expressed by the specialist – is confirmed and formalized.

I started this study by asking why patients with a small-cell lung carcinoma are so optimistic about recovery. I discovered that they are particularly optimistic in the remission phase. Patients do not hope for a cure, which is why I avoid the term 'hope' in favour of 'optimism,' but they do believe they will recover. The optimism develops during first-line chemotherapy and is supported by the X-rays, which show clear remission, and by the doctor's positive words. This optimism gradually breaks down after the phase of remission, both as result of the patient's own experience (the

3 For example in the case of Mr Dekker in Chapter 1.

tumour recurs) and the doctor's reaction to this ('this is a normal development for this kind of cancer'). However, due to the optimism experienced during first-line therapy and the doctor's positive feedback, the patient generally chooses to undergo second-line therapy. During this phase he is again optimistic, but to a lesser extent. One difference compared with the first treatment is that the optimism now is not unambiguously supported by the X-rays and the doctor's words. In this way the patient gradually learns more about his illness, and he collaborates with the specialist in working towards the denouement.

Even when optimism is the dominant mood, it is not the only emotion; there is also fear, desperation and anxiety. During the whole course of the illness patients have to deal with feelings of uncertainty. However, during both the stage of desperation and that of optimism, the patient is still largely unaware of what the doctor knows. And this is because he is not clearly and repeatedly told.

Long-term and short-term perspectives

In the previous section I might have given the impression that specialists only provide their patients with information on one or two occasions during the 1–2 year course of the illness. In fact, doctors are continually informing patients about their current situation and about short-term treatment options. This information is, however, of a different kind from that relating to the general prognosis of the illness and the fatal outcome, i.e. the long-term perspective. The 'change of course' from fatal diagnosis to treatment that takes place during the first bad news interview is maintained during treatment and remission. During check-ups conversation is limited almost exclusively to the short-term aspects of treatment such as side effects of the chemotherapy, laboratory results, instructions, making treatment as comfortable as possible, planning further appointments, etc. The short-term perspective is dependent on the long-term perspective. The general course of the illness is what is likely to happen based on probabilities ('this is how lung carcinoma generally develops'). The short-term perspective is fixed (chemotherapy follows a standard protocol), but if the long-term perspective changes (the tumour progresses in spite of therapy) then the short-term perspective is adjusted accordingly (chemotherapy is stopped and other treatment is initiated).

Costain Schou (1993, 1999) has also noted that specialists continually focus on the short-term and do not discuss the long-term aspects of the illness. Into the patient's existential uncertainty the doctor introduces order, occupying his time with activities (treatment, check-ups) and suggestions of certainty (treatment schemes, laboratory tests). Specialists inform their patients mainly about these fixed aspects of treatment, and this diverts the patient's attention from the more general uncertainties of his condition.[4] De Swaan (1985) also notes that specialists seldom discuss the long-term perspective of illness. He describes clearly how specialists render statements about the long-term perspective and prognosis dependent on the short-term perspective. They give their patients the impression that they can only really say anything about prognosis once they know how the treatment is working. However, when the time arrives they again postpone explanation and make it dependent on future treatment and further tests. Although de Swaan fails to describe the phased way in which doctors inform their patients, and his descriptions of doctors' actions are rather strategically oriented, he does appositely describe the essence of the process. Because the patient is continually promised something, he never really has the chance to prepare for death (de Swaan 1985: 19). The advantage of the short-term perspective is that it gives the patient the opportunity to avoid thinking about the disastrous outcome of his illness and allows him to concentrate on the near future. The short-term perspective structures the illness process for the patient and his relatives and renders this difficult period orderly and manageable. De Swaan goes as far as to claim that treatment has a sedative effect in itself (de Swaan 1985).

It was striking how doctors answered patients' questions about the long-term perspective of their illness in terms of the short-term perspective. Maguire and Faulkner (1988a, b) claims that when patients raise psychological and medical complaints, doctors and nurses tend to concentrate only on the medical issues. He calls this reaction, which he thinks is an unconscious one, the 'distancing technique'. Focusing on the medical aspects of patients' problems and distancing themselves from their psychological suffering enables doctors and nurses to cope emotionally. While I agree with Maguire's analysis, I also think that doctors' and nurses' interpretation of their role is an important factor. In various parts of this book it is clear that specialists concentrate on the medical-technical aspects of treatment; that is where their expertise and responsibility lie. When non-clinical factors are involved, medical specialists tend to consider this the domain of others, such as relatives, nurses, social workers, and GPs. There is some individual variation, of course, and while many specialists see their role as strictly medical-technical, some do ascribe themselves a more psychosocial role.[5] Moreover, the extent of psychosocial support given by the specialist varies from one

---

4 Costain Schou (1993) has implicitly discussed the short and long-term aspects of illness, and my results support her analysis. However, I prefer the terms 'short-term perspective' and 'long-term perspective' to her 'calendar' and 'trajectory' because I want to emphasize the temporal aspect.
5 The lung specialist in training Ilona Racz and Dorien Meulman, for example, think that psycho-social support is part of their job.

patient to another.[6] This narrowing of the doctor's role is part of the general development in health care, with its increasing specialization and super specialization.

De Swaan (1985) describes how all participants – patients, specialists, and nurses – are interdependent in the apportioning of attention in the hospital's emotional economy. This attention has three aspects: medical care, information and support. Patients demand more attention than doctors can provide, and in this sense attention is a scarce commodity. It is the task of doctors and nurses to respond to the patient's physical complaints. This is particularly so in the case of the patients in this study, when even apparently minor symptoms may point to a recurrent tumour. As a result, physical complaints are almost always taken seriously and investigated. According to de Swaan, the physical aspect of the illness and its medical treatment are not simply the most important factors but often the *only* important ones in the hospital (de Swaan 1985: 30, 35). When patients become aware of how the system works, they adjust, and when they somatize their psychosocial problems they are assured of the doctor's attention. In this way the need for attention is made technical and a process of somatization and medicalization is set in motion. The system is self-perpetuating; in a totally medicalized context the focus of specialists on the physical and medical aspects of illness and treatment is to be expected.

The concepts of a short- and a long-term perspective enable me to express what I found most striking about the communication process I studied: the disproportionate amount of time spent – by both doctors and patients – on relatively trivial matters. In doing so I want to emphasize the contrast between large, long-term problems (the incurable illness that will soon kill the patient in spite of treatment) and the relatively small short-term problems relating to treatment. This is undoubtedly related to the strongly felt need in western culture for control and the related tendency to regard all problems as controllable and solvable. And from this stems the tendency to fragment problems we do not want to confront because we cannot solve them. From large problems we make smaller ones, which are solvable, or at any rate manageable. Because of our problem solving optimism, we transform the dying trajectory into fragments that are emotionally convenient.

In spite of their concentration on the here-and-now of treatment, patients do, in the course of their illness, develop their own view of the long-term

---

6 This is because the relationship between a doctor and his patient and the patient's partner vary. Dr Liem did not really consider the provision of psycho-social support to be one of his tasks. But in spite of this it was possible to observe differences from one patient to another. For example, during the final stages of her husband's illness, he allowed Mrs Wessels to call him on an almost daily basis for emotional support. Here individual factors played a role: Dr Liem knew that they could not rely on the GP and that Mrs Wessels had trouble coping with her husband's illness.

perspective. They learn from the changing medical situation and interpret verbal and non-verbal information relating to their illness. They also *go in search* of evidence. One strategy is to ask questions such as, 'I won't make Christmas, will I?' My research has shown how important the context of fellow-patients is in this quest for information about the general trajectory and prognosis of the illness. From the very beginning, in the waiting room and ward, patients closely and fearfully observe those who share their fate. They compare themselves to other patients and gradually build up a picture of the course their illness is likely to take (Costain Schou 1993: 250). When the specialist's messages are positive and they receive positive images from other patients – such as during first-line chemotherapy and remission – patients identify strongly with one another. They see in others evidence that 'all will end well'. When their fellow patients are not doing so well, two opposing processes become visible. The first is that the patient distances himself from the fate of other patients by emphasizing the differences ('He's got metastases in his liver and bones, mine are only in my head').[7] The second is that the patient identifies with his fellow patient and his situation and recognizes it as a taste of what is to come (rehearsal).[8] These two processes are not independent. In this book I have shown how the total process of identification and distancing works, and how patients in different phases of their illness alternate between seeking support and distancing themselves from fellow patients.

Public information and hidden information

When, after not having seen her for a long time, I ran into Liesbeth Quint, one of the patients in my study, I only just managed to hide my surprise that she was still alive. This made me realize the extent of the contrast between the 'hidden' discussions in which I participated as an outsider and in which patients' prognoses were discussed openly, and the veiled nature of the communication with the patient. I suddenly became aware that it was possible to distinguish between a *public* short-term perspective and a *hidden* long-term perspective.

I call the information about the long-term perspective 'hidden' because the doctor only discusses it with the patient at certain points in the illness trajectory, mostly during the bad news interview, and otherwise only in response to the patient's repeated questioning. Among themselves, however, doctors and nurses *do* talk openly about the long-term perspective

---

7 I have mentioned earlier that doctors try to reassure patients by individualizing their disease process.
8 This term is from Glaser and Strauss 1965.

and the patient's prognosis. By contrast, the information about the short-term of the illness is 'public,' that is it is available for everyone and anyone can discuss it freely with the patient at any time. Doctors are continually and voluntarily informing their patients about this aspect of their illness and do not avoid patients' questions about it.

Patients are therefore confronted with two conflicting discourses (Britten 1991). On the one hand there is an 'open' discourse in which they are told about their treatment and allowed to look at X-rays, CT scans and laboratory results. In relation to the short-term perspective they are treated as autonomous individuals. On the other hand, when it comes to the long-term prognosis, doctors become more paternalistic and protective.

As a result of my meeting with Liesbeth Quint, I realized that the problems that nurses have in communicating with patients relate to the long-term and not the short-term perspective. Nurses did not interfere in the information exchange between doctors and patients regarding the long-term of the illness. However, if a patient was uncertain about a treatment schedule, then they did not hesitate to consult the treatment protocol and inform him.[9] If, on the other hand, a patient cherished hopes of cure or expressed unrealistic plans for the future, the nurses tended not to contradict this. The nurses could also look this information up, but they did not, because this would conflict with the dominant code according to which the specialist is the initiator and source of long-term information about the illness (Kellehear 1992). Both doctors and nurses agree that it is the specialist (in charge of that patient) who should be the first to inform him about the general course of his illness. Others – other doctors, but especially nurses – can only speak of such matters with the specialist's permission, and they have to adjust what they say to what he has or has not told the patient (de Swaan 1985: 32).

The problem for nurses in the outpatient clinic is that they are not present when the doctor discusses the long-term perspective with the patient. When patients are on the ward, the nurses are represented during bad news interviews, but this does not solve the general communication problem. Most of the bad news interviews take place in the outpatient clinic, as does most of the treatment and follow-up of patients. Outpatient clinic nurses do not have any direct way of knowing what the patient knows about his illness, and so are not sure how to relate what they say to what the patient knows. The specialist may say that he has told the patient 'everything,' but if the patient shows no sign of this knowledge then the nurses can only guess. This is why nurses attempt, throughout the illness trajectory, to find

---

9 This openness with regard to the short-term perspective also has a practical dimension: if patients were not informed about the short-term details it would be impossible to get them to come to the hospital for treatment (Costain Schou 1993, 1999).

out what exactly the patient knows. Even if the specialist or the patient gives a detailed account of the bad news interview, uncertainty remains. The import of the choice of words, use of pauses, exchange of meaningful glances, is difficult to replicate. Moreover, those involved – doctor and patient – often have different interpretations of what was said, and they will repeat these interpretations when giving their account of the discussion. An important aspect of this is that many patients *want* to get better and this in turn affects the extent to which they allow medical reality to impinge on their perceptions. They hear only what they want to hear and interpret that information in a manner that is acceptable to them.

There are various reasons why the information relating to the long-term perspective is important for the nurses. The nurses' relationship with patients differs from that of doctors. Providing psychosocial support is an important aspect of the nurses' job. If they knew more about the communication during the bad news interview they would feel less awkward and have more freedom of expression in their discussions with patients. This would not only improve communication between patient and nurse, but also facilitate the task of the specialist. The distinction between public information about the short-term perspective and hidden information about the long-term perspective makes it easier to understand the tensions between nurses and specialists that I encountered at the beginning of this study. The nurses wonder whether the specialist has been truthful to the patient, that is whether he has informed the patient about the long-term perspective. The specialist says that he has 'discussed everything openly with the patient,' referring to what he has said about the short-term perspective. I have already mentioned what Maguire refers to as the 'distancing technique'. De Swaan also noticed a process of medicalization and somatization in the specialist cancer hospital in which he carried out his research. Both these authors describe a tendency among both doctors and nurses to prioritize patients' short-term somatic complaints while at the same time ignoring other, non-somatic, problems. In my research I only encountered this tendency among the doctors. If it was simply a matter of distancing then why did the nurses in this study not make use of this tactic. Many of the nurses in my study criticized the doctors for this very focus on the somatic domain, while at the same time trying to devote attention to the patients' psychosocial needs. Indeed, the nurses seemed to claim this latter domain as their own and define psychosocial support as one of their tasks.

The reason for this difference between my results and those of Maguire and de Swaan is not difficult to find. De Swaan did his research during the 1970s, Maguire during the early 1980s. My study was carried out in the 1990s. During the intervening years nurses have developed and defined different goals for themselves as a professional group. New, more theoretically oriented curricula have been developed to train nurses, and more time is devoted to the psychosocial aspects of their work. I noticed a clear difference between nurses who had an in-service training and those who had been trained externally: the latter were much more critical about the communication between doctors and patients while the former were more focused on practical everyday tasks. The nurses themselves shared this perception. Nurses in charge generally tried to achieve a balanced representation of both groups in their teams.

Ambiguity and the hope of a cure

The communication I have been discussing is also characterized by many different forms of ambiguity. In this section I focus on ambiguity in the treatment context, how patients interpret this and the resulting hope of recovery. In discussions about the long-term perspective of the illness, specialists are often careful about what they say, and their choice of words is often ambiguous. To a certain extent this ambiguity is unintentional. For example, the connotations of the word 'to treat' (*behandelen*) are more positive in every day use than they are in a clinical context. If a doctor says, 'the tumour is treatable,' then the patient interprets this as meaning that something can be done, that 'things will be okay,' whereas the clinical interpretation is more neutral, implying 'action' (*handelen*) or 'doing' (*doen*). However, this ambiguity can also be conscious. The specialist who says to the patient after chemotherapy, 'there are no longer any abnormalities visible on the X-ray,' or 'your lungs are clear,' is telling the truth. However, the patient, who is unaware of the general trajectory of his illness, will interpret this as cure. I call this ambiguity conscious because, although the specialist does not actually tell the patient that he is cured, he is aware that this is how the patient interprets his statement, and he makes no attempt to prevent this misinterpretation.

The term 'chemo*therapy*' is also ambiguous in this context. In everyday usage, 'therapy' has as its expected outcome 'cure'. In the case of small-cell lung carcinoma, however, the term is being used to refer to an *incurable* illness. The term 'therapy' is used in this sense in the context of other incurable illnesses, such as diabetes and certain infectious diseases, but there are important differences. Small-cell lung carcinoma patients and diabetics are both incurably ill, but the cancer patients will all die in the very short-term, whereas the diabetics will not. The term therapy is more acceptable when applied to diabetics because treatment serves to prevent the condition from becoming worse, and with therapy the patient generally still has a long life to look forward to. In the case of small-cell lung carcinoma the goal of therapy is palliative and the extension of the patient's life is only for a few months, or one or two years at most. Specialists know, from the very beginning, that the patient with small-cell lung carcinoma will die in the short-term, in spite of treatment, and yet they speak of 'therapy'. It may seem somewhat exaggerated to dwell on the semantics of these terms, but it is useful because it tells us something about doctors' (unconscious) desire to cure.[10]

Moreover, there are also conscious and unconscious *non-verbal* ambiguities. For example, patients with small-cell lung carcinoma are treated so intensively that it is hard for them to imagine that all this effort is for 'nothing,' i.e. that it does not result in cure. Specialists do say that their efforts are palliative and meant to extend the patient's life for as long as possible, but their actions nonetheless give a curative impression. To some extent this occurs independently of the intentions of the individual doctor. Public emphasis on cure, and socially propagated optimism about the potential of medical science play an important role in this. In the media, and in the information provided by health care institutions, the emphasis is on the success of medical interventions, rather than on the failures and the impossibilities. This image created expectations among patients and gives the impression that solutions can be found for all health problems.

I have described how the response of the tumour to chemotherapy as seen on the X-rays stimulates the patient's optimism. The doctors are also sensitive to this, however. One of the doctors once remarked that when he saw that the tumour had 'disappeared' from the X-ray, the thought did cross his mind that perhaps the impossible had really happened. Specialists must cherish some (unconscious) hope that their patient will be cured, and it is possible that during treatment it is not only the hope of the patient that is at stake. It is not only the patient who is in a difficult situation, but also the doctor treating him. During consultation the specialist informs a patient that he is going to die and 15 minutes later he is with the next patient. Obviously doctors identify and empathize with the patient, and to a greater or lesser extent the specialist is confronted with his own attitudes to life and death, with his own emotions and mortality.[11] By fighting for the patient and not depriving him of hope, the specialist not only gives the patient courage to face his illness, but also keeps his own hope alive. This hope is not only focused on the short-term, but especially on the long-term. During my research I came to realize that this hope is related to clinical trials. Trials not only have scientific goals, they also generate meaning.

Then there is the recurrent dilemma of optimism versus fear: 'How often should you repeat to the patient that he is not going to get better? Should you keep knocking him down with this information?' one doctor asked. De

---

10 Another illustration of this desire to cure is the way they refer to the results of treating a disease with such a poor prognosis as the *survival* rate.
11 This does not apply only to doctors, of course, but to all those working in a health-care setting, especially for the nurses who are much 'closer' to the patients than the doctors.

Swaan has argued that specialists' statements that the patient's hope has a positive effect on the disease process result in patients believing that their mental and emotional disposition and their perseverance can have a positive influence on their cancer (de Swaan 1985: 37). I was often struck by patients' truculence and the doggedness, as though any improvement was solely of their own doing. Patients often viewed their illness as a personal crusade, something that they could win through struggle. When they saw the favourable results on the X-ray, patients often exclaimed that they had 'done their best' or 'maintained a positive attitude'.

The specialists have, to a significant extent, given the patients with small-cell lung carcinoma the hope that they cherish. First, during the bad news interview the doctor tells the patient that he is sick when he does not feel sick at all. Then, during the period of treatment and remission the patient generally feels sicker than at the point of diagnosis (partly due to the treatment itself) but the specialist now says that things are 'going well'. In various respects patients are 'abandoned' by their bodies. Not only is their body sick, but that body no longer tells them clearly 'how they are doing'. It is no longer the patient himself who feels how he is doing, but the doctor who tells him. In the case of small-cell lung carcinoma X-rays play a determinant role in this. With these the specialist can illustrate and prove his statements, even if they are the opposite of what the patient feels. As their illness progresses, patients become increasingly dependent on the specialist, and his words are given added significance (de Swaan 1985). If the specialist says that things are okay then they are okay. When I spoke to patients just before an outpatient clinic check-up and asked them how they were they often shrugged. They were nervous and did not know. They could only answer my question after they had seen the doctor. However, it is not only the patients who attach so much significance to the doctors' words. Friends and relatives are generally also more interested in the specialist's evaluation of how the patient is than in what the patient himself says. This dependency is particularly clear in the case of seriously ill patients who are about to die. In life-threatening situations the drive to survive becomes more pronounced and people are more inclined to orient themselves to the doctor.

Nurses and GPs resist this encouragement of hope of a cure in patients. It is understandable why these professions are critical. The specialist is the author of this hope, and the other involved professions have to collaborate. Moreover, nurses and GPs do not participate in the communication between specialist and patient.[12] The dissatisfaction is related to the way in

---

12 In this respect their position is similar to that of the researcher. The nurses were struck by patients' unjustified optimism much more than the specialists, just as I was. The difference is that I was later able to distance myself from this.

which patients spend this final phase of their life. They are immersed in a clinical world, in which it is difficult to choose any other narrative than that of tests, treatment and related hope of cure. Nurses (and GPs) experience most difficulty with the fact that patients are not supported in their quest for what would be, for them, a good death. The obsession with treatment and the hope of cure – by both specialist and patient – obscure other narratives (Frank 1995: 83). Nurses and GPs often have other ideas about how the final stage of the patient's life should be spent. Their frustration is that they are closely involved in the care of the patient but do not have the means to place the dying patient's experience in any other context than that of the clinical narrative mentioned above.

It is important to realize that taking away patients' hope of cure does not deprive them of all hope. In my discussions with patients I have seen other forms of hope survive. For example, Mr van der Velde hoped to see the opening of his son's new law firm, and the Wessels family hoped to be able to share an Indonesian meal on Mr Wessels's birthday. Mr Dekker hoped to retain his identity and his personality up until the end, and he hoped that his loved ones would remember him in this way (see also Nuland 1995). This brings me to another form of powerlessness that confronts those who deal with the incurably ill and the dying. Van Dantzig describes how the tendency of doctors to talk to patients in a comforting way increases as the patient's misery increases (Gelauff and Manschot 1997: 201). In the Dutch culture, to comfort is generally interpreted as 'speaking in a consoling manner'. According to Van Dantzig, comfort can also mean the recognition that the other is having a hard time, including all the related feelings of sadness, fear, anger and jealousy. This recognition can assist in helping patients to find ways – 'real' solutions – to confront the reality of death (Nuland 1995).

The restitution narrative and other stories

Patients' optimism is not only a result of communication, and it is not only developed by the doctors, but also by the patients themselves. Is this optimism really a characteristic of the patient, or is it socially generated, with the patient simply clinging to it in the hope that 'everything will be all right'? Above I discussed the socially desirable 'restitution narrative'. In fact, the illness trajectory of the patient is influenced by a number of narratives.

In his book, *The Wounded Storyteller*, Frank discussed the 'restitution narrative' extensively. He describes how, in our culture, it is socially desirable that patients tell restitution narratives. We want to hear this narrative from patients; when we hear others we are often unsure how to react. Whether we are watching a serious documentary about health care or a television soap opera, reading a hospital brochure or a newspaper article about illness, the storyline is: yesterday the person was healthy, today he is sick, but tomorrow he will be better, thanks to medical science. The bare bones of the storyline are fleshed out with details of laboratory tests, treatment, discoveries, clinical expertise and, often, a contribution by the patient. The restitution plot dominates most patients' narratives, especially those of patients who have recently fallen ill (Frank 1995: 83).

Many patients do recover, and for them the restitution narrative is appropriate. Patients with a small-cell lung carcinoma do not get better, and here we reach the limits of the restitution narrative: people are mortal. Death has no place in these narratives. In Part IV, I described how patients kept expressing optimism in the final phase of life. I struggled trying to understand how obviously dying patients could insist that they were going to recover. I could hardly believe that these patients and their loved ones really believed these increasingly unbelievable statements, but I could not confront them with my disbelief. If they did not believe these stories, why did they tell them? In his book Frank wonders what happens to patients who have the courage to discuss their approaching death. What is left for people, who have always talked in terms of recovery, to tell when they have left behind all hope of recovery? According to Frank, the tragedy is not so much death itself, but that the narrative that the patient himself so enthusiastically and persistently pronounced, has ended before his life has finished. The patient is still alive, but has 'nothing more to say'. Patients generally have difficulty telling any other narrative than the restitution narrative. Frank describes how patients are expected to recover from their illnesses (Frank 1995). The restitution narrative not only reflects the 'natural' desire of the patient to get better, patients have also *learned* to tell them.

The restitution narrative is particularly important early on in the illness. I have described how, after the desperation following diagnosis and the concomitant existential crisis, patients then surrender and focus on treatment. In the remission phase the restitution narrative seems to be unambiguously confirmed, and it becomes appropriate to use. In this phase patients really believe in recovery. With the return of the tumour, the deterioration of fellow patients and the less hopeful statements of the specialists, the patient becomes anxious and doubts about the restitution narrative surface. But by then it is difficult to retract. It is always difficult to admit you were wrong. This is particularly true in the case of the restitution narrative. This is because, as I have described, hope of cure is a *collective* rather than an individual phenomenon.[13] When a patient creates restitution narrative together with his loved ones, it is difficult for him to unilaterally reject it. Patients use narratives strategically, they have the 'duty' towards the other 'authors' to stick to the story. Patients and their relatives may also keep the

---

13 See Chapter 5.

narrative going in order to protect each other. Sometimes this protection is one-sided.[14] I sometimes had the impression that this was particularly the case with patients whose relatives accompanied them to the hospital less frequently. These relatives were more dependent on the patient for their information. Another example of this one-sided protection is when parents try to protect their unknowing or more positively inclined children. Sometimes both patient and relatives attempt to protect each other, and the narrative of cure is mutually kept alive.[15] Those involved try to act as 'normally' as possible and to be brave, while knowing deep down inside that things are not as they should be.[16] Usually both sides claim that they are coping with the situation but do not want to talk about it in order to protect the other.[17]

It is striking that a few of the more highly educated patients in this study did not make use of restitution narratives; they seemed to understand and accept clinical reality sooner. Partly as a result of this, the specialists were more open with them. The interesting question here is whether these patients were really less optimistic. It is also possible that their reason for not using these narratives was not so much that they did not believe them, but that their social environment would not have accepted them, that the patient would have been *forced* to accept the truth. Something similar happened in the case of Mrs Rogge. She tended toward optimism but this was countered by her social environment. Each time she made an optimistic statement her children would remind her of the clinical reality of her situation. The restitution narrative is perhaps not as universal as Frank assumes.

Apart from the fact that I did not understand how patients who were obviously deteriorating rapidly could persist in their optimism about the possibility of recovery, I was also often confused by the inconsistency of their statements. One moment I was confronted with optimism, the next with desperation. What was the *truth*? It took some time before I realized that when I saw only the restitution narrative I was not getting below the surface. Further analysis revealed that patients and their relatives do not only have a single narrative; they use *multiple narratives* simultaneously, and all are equally true for them. Patients therefore do not simply use narratives for strategic reasons, they also believe them.

In previous research I discovered how differently patients express themselves depending on to whom they are talking (The 1996, 1997a, 1998).

---

14 It is possible that patients also tried to protect me. As the research proceeded I had an increasingly close bond with the patients.
15 For example Mr de Jager in Chapter 10.
16 Nuland (1995) and Frank (1995) give excellent examples of this.
17 Only 54 per cent of the patients in Kellehear's study (1992: 78) shared with a partner the realization that they were dying.

Tensions regularly arose between doctors and nurses relating to patients' euthanasia requests. The most common pattern was that the nurses interpreted a request as 'genuine' whereas the doctors did not. This was because the patients talked about these issues differently from doctors and nurses. Euthanasia was more likely to be discussed when talking to the nurses. Initially I thought that this was because communication with the nurses was easier to initiate because they were more accessible, that patients who really want euthanasia tend to say this to the nurses. Later on I noticed that they were ambivalent: that sometimes they really wanted euthanasia and sometimes they really did not. When they think about the suffering and the fatal outcome of their illness they want to die as soon as possible to avoid this. On the other hand, when they think of all the things they love and do not want to miss, then they cling to life. So they talk to the nurses about euthanasia during moments when they want to die, but not to the doctors who actually make the decisions about granting euthanasia request. When a patient hears that the tumour has disappeared, when he thinks back to how he struggled to complete treatment and realizes that the victory was well earned, when he sees fellow patients in the waiting room, apparently happy and glowing with health, then the restitution narrative is real and justified. When the same patient lies awake at night worrying about the pain in his chest, what the doctor could have meant by certain remarks, what the future holds then the desperation – I call this the desperation narrative – is also real and justified. Depending on the context and the situation one of the narratives is appropriate and true. Truth for the patient is not unequivocal. This is why their optimism can vary depending on whether they are with doctors or nurses.

Patients possess a register of *different* narratives that, although they may be contradictory, are nonetheless all genuine (Glaser and Strauss 1965). And it is not only terminal patients who utilize different narratives. Everyone lives with various narratives and it is a constant struggle to create unity between these narratives, to create unity in one's life. This is a characteristic of life, but it is particularly pertinent at the end of life. In order to achieve closure it is important for patients to introduce some degree of unity in these diverse narratives, but it is unclear whether they have sufficient chance to do this. This failure is due not only to illness and death but – as I have attempted to show – to various related factors. The restitution narrative – composed from the doctor's words, the patient's will to recover, his reluctance to know the truth, the ambiguities of the situation and the more general social restitution narrative – is dominant. As a result there is a temptation to see only the patient's optimism. The restitution narrative is told; the patient's fear, anxiety and worries are suffered in silence. This is why I initially saw only the restitution narrative, later noticed the desperation narrative and finally realized that both were interwoven into a single reality.

The latent realization of approaching death

Both recovery and desperation narratives coexist throughout the patient's illness trajectory, although they alternate in their relevance from one stage of the illness to another. Closely related to this is the patient's latent realization of his approaching death, which I will consider in this section.

The clinical trajectory of the illness and the gradual realization of death were not always synchronic in the patients I studied. Usually the patient's realization lagged behind the clinical progression of his illness; sometimes the realization was overtaken by the rapid progression of the illness, but it develops gradually in most patients. First they lose their optimism; they realize they are going to die but are not sure when,[18] and this is the long-term perspective that specialists present to their patients. Although the realization of death develops gradually, it does not generally proceed through a series of phases. Rather there is, in both patient and relatives, a *latent realization* (Sheehy 1973). Depending on the context, it might be in the foreground one minute and hardly perceptible the next (Kellehear 1992).

The latent realization of death is accompanied by ambivalence. On the one hand patients seem to comprehend the truth, but at the same time they do not. I was surprised that patients and their relatives never got angry when, shortly before the patient's death, the specialist dashed any remaining hope by placing clinical reality firmly in the forefront. I had thought that, when they realized that their optimism was based on an illusion, patients would blame the specialist for creating and maintaining this illusion. This may be due to loyalty or continuing dependence, but that is not the only reason. Patients and their relatives usually listened to the specialist's words calmly. They sounded sincere when they replied that they had 'really known all along' and that 'the doctor had made the situation clear,' but that it had not sunk in because it was so incredible. Patients seem to find themselves in a situation of simultaneously knowing and not knowing. Their calm reaction to the revelation, at the end of their illness trajectory, that their optimism had been unjustified, is explained partly by the fact that they had possessed the latent knowledge of their demise from the start. Because of this latent realization, the ambivalence, the defence mechanisms, the competing narratives, and the need to share the understanding with others, it is difficult to discover exactly what a patient knows about the long-term perspective of his illness (Kellehear 1992).

I have already discussed the hidden long-term perspective and the public short-term perspective, but I have not yet considered why they exist simultaneously. It is much more difficult for specialists to talk to patients about

---

18 Glaser and Strauss (1965) discuss this in an 'open realization' context. Here I would note that realization that you are dying does not necessarily mean acceptance of death.

the long-term than about the short-term aspects of the illness. Lack of time, courage, and emotional resources result in the specialist avoiding discussion of the long-term. Moreover, it is tempting to offer desperate patients comfort and solutions (see Gelauff and Manschot 1997: 201). I agree with Costain Schou that there is a gap between the modern ideals of openness and truth and reality, in which there is insufficient time and opportunity to put them into practice (Costain Schou 1993: 252).

According to the modern democratic ideology of openness and self-determination it is good for patients to be completely aware of and have a say in what is going on. The problem is that patients – and people generally – do not want to know about and have a say in difficult and fundamental issues. The point I made earlier, about patients interpreting the positive information that specialists give them about the short-term as information about the long-term, could also be interpreted in this way. Patients enquire about the long-term perspective, but they only want to hear positive answers. The idea of a 'latent' realization suggests that the patient does know while at the same time not wanting to know. I have said much about the ambiguous context in which the patient receives treatment. What should not be forgotten, however, is that patients maintain this ambiguity as long as it is convenient for them. For them, knowing and not knowing are functional. I have already remarked a number of times that specialists 'follow' the extent of patients' realization. It is quite possible that they adjust their communication with patients to take this into account. Outsiders tend to think that specialists flout the rules and simply do what is convenient for themselves. The maintenance of the patient's optimism about cure is then often blamed – as I initially did myself – on the specialist's reluctance to be honest. During the course of my research I came to the conclusion that patients have much more control over the discourse relating to the long-term of their illness that is initially apparent. This means that the existing system of communication is more attuned to the needs of the patient than it appears.

This brings me to a rather different conclusion about the communication between doctors and patients than I had anticipated at the start of my study. It leads me to question just how great the achievements of the modern age really are. I do not have the answer. In the past, when doctors kept the medical truth from their patients, uncertainty and fear were tempered by ignorance. If patients did suspect, then they could turn to religion. In the modern secular age with its ideal of openness, the patient finds himself in a void. There is no more blind faith in medicine and no religion to mitigate the final realization of impending death. *Honesty* and *facing the truth* are the ideals, but many patients are unable to cope with them, even those who are highly educated. Take the father of the GP van Zomeren for example. This ex-GP had witnessed the deaths of many patients, but when his son informed him of his approaching end, he did not want to face the truth. Such examples make one wonder whether the old system might have been better. I exchanged e-mails about this with Robert Pool and at one point he wrote, 'What has become clear to me after studying traditional medicine in both India and Africa, is the importance – the healing and soothing effect – of the belief in the infallibility of the healer. It does not matter that this belief is objectively untenable; it is religious. Traditional medicine 'works' because people believe it will work. Sometimes, during my own research in the hospital,[19] I thought that some of the patients would have died a "better" death if they had been given less of the truth (e.g. not been shown exactly how large the tumour had become on the X-ray) and more of what they really wanted to hear. Somewhere deep inside they know that they are going to die, why does it have to be made so conscious and explicit. Maybe this is all part of Dutch sobriety.'

Patients need something other than the ideal of openness and self-determination that we hold up to them and to ourselves. The patients in this study did not always want to know everything and have everything made explicit. What they wanted was care and attention for themselves, their social environment and the consequences that their illness has for their lives. But that is not all. Patients also experience the need to talk and to tell in their own – non-medical – terms. Because what patients and their relatives need does not have a high priority in the medical world, there is little opportunity to fulfil these needs. During this study I was sometimes poignantly aware of the gap between the patients' needs and clinical practice; I regularly had the impression that doctors and patients were on completely different wavelengths. This relationship between doctors and patients was not the only complexity, however. External factors also played a role. In the next two sections I turn to these factors; I will examine 'choice' and discuss some related legal issues.

'Choosing' treatment

Choice, Mol writes, has in recent years rapidly been transformed into an ideal. 'Firstly within professional action itself. At present, most attempts to improve the quality of care are aimed at doctors. If doctors made more rational choices and provided more support for their calculations, then this would lead to an improvement in care, or so it is thought. Meanwhile, ethicists, jurists and patient activists point to the possibility of allowing patients to make decisions in which values are at issue. After all, care is all

---

19 Robert Pool studied euthanasia decisions in the 'Randstad Hospital' in the Netherlands (see Pool 2000).

about their lives. That is why it is better that patients, who have been given adequate information, choose themselves' (Mol 1997a: 3, my translation). Earlier I remarked that choice is especially important for those who are receiving palliative care. Doctors determine whether a treatment is medically feasible, but it is only the patient (and his close family and friends) who can take the non-medical decision as to whether the treatment is meaningful for him. The doctor's expertise stems from his profession, the patient's from his life; each has his own responsibility (Kompanje 1998: 21). I assumed that self-determination and autonomy were appropriate *par excellence* in palliative care. I have already discussed communication and information provision in the case of patients with a small-cell lung carcinoma. In what follows I will discuss the way in which decisions about treatment are taken during the whole illness trajectory.

There are two characteristic aspects of the decision process relating to patients with small-cell lung carcinoma. Firstly, due to the explosive growth of the tumour, treatment has to start almost immediately and so there is not much time in which to make the necessary decisions. Secondly, during the one or two years of their illness, patients are repeatedly confronted with the choice of whether or not to let themselves be treated. The patients in this study were surprisingly homogenous in their decisions: agreeing to treatment was the only possible choice. Overwhelmed by events and without medical knowledge, patients immediately agreed with the treatment suggested by the specialist. They hardly ever made a choice that deviated from what the doctor proposed. Caught between fear and inflated expectations of the outcome of therapy, they accepted what was offered without hesitation. They hardly ever asked questions about the proposed treatment or possible alternatives. During consultations the advantages and disadvantages of therapy were not discussed extensively. Patients did not seem to attach much importance to the side effects of treatment, which the doctor dutifully enumerated; they were waved aside and accepted in advance. Although this appears to be a crucial decision, patients almost never needed extra time to think, discuss the decision with others or get advice. On the contrary, most patients wanted to be treated as soon as possible – 'today rather than tomorrow'. They often only calmed down when 'something was being done'. When asked why they chose to be treated, all patients answered that they 'had no choice'. They claimed to have their 'back against the wall' (Wagener 1987: 1007). 'Doing nothing,' waiting at home for the end, was not an option. They all wanted to grasp the chance that was being offered and try the therapy. They were afraid that they would later regret it if they 'had not made the effort.'[20]

---

20 Tijmstra describes the process of 'anticipated decision regret'. Patients decide to accept therapy because they anticipate that that they will regret it if they do not.

Although healthy people usually claim that they would definitely want to participate in the decision process if they were ill, when they actually fall sick this turns out not to be the case. The shock caused by the bad news can eliminate any desire to participate (Degner and Sloan 1992). Disease, exhaustion, pain, fear and discomfort, all experienced in the overwhelming context of the hospital, fundamentally influence the patient's resistance (Kompanje 1998: 30–1). This decline in the desire to participate in the decision process seems to be particularly pronounced in those with serious fatal illnesses (Ende et al. 1989). Such patients are often no longer capable of participation. The sick would rather hand over control to someone else; their need is more for care, relief and support (Nuland 1995). In fact, this is only to be expected. 'Don't the sick need care?' Mol asks. 'That is why they come to care providers in the first place. It is inappropriate to say to them, 'You tell us what you want us to do'. That ignores the fact that the various possibilities in the specific situation of the sick individual are often too complex to oversee readily. Who, whether they are sick or healthy, can think in terms of possibilities, percentages, risks and chances of success? Isn't that what the doctor is supposed to do for you?' (Mol 1997a: 145, my translation). In most cases patients do not come to the doctor with the intention of taking part in the decisions; they come for solutions to their health problems, to be cured, to receive treatment and care (Verheggen 1996: 122). Most patients with a serious, fatal illness are confused and hardly capable of overseeing their situation. In order to be able to choose, Mol argues, the individual must be capable of and willing to make the choice; he must have learned how to insert himself into the process of choosing and he must have developed the necessary abilities (Mol 1997b), such as the ability to weigh the different interests that are involved. Many of the patients in my study felt that they could not choose, and therefore shifted the responsibility back to the specialist. They want 'something' to be done as soon as possible and when the specialist proposes a course of treatment they answer, 'What would you do?' or 'You do what you think is best.'

First-line chemotherapy was hardly ever refused. I discussed in Part I how the exceptional refusal is rooted in the biography of the individual patient. The refusals in this study were based on the extensive experience of the treatment of incurable cancer patients (see Chapter 1). All those who refused therapy knew that it was not curative and they belonged to the small minority of patients who were not optimistic about recovery. However, not all patients who were not optimistic refused treatment. Of the three patients who were obviously not optimistic about recovery and who accepted therapy, two had higher education. This was striking because all the others were not highly educated. In the case of the third patient, her children – who worked in health care – refused to accept her optimism.

All those who had accepted first-line chemotherapy also accepted second-line therapy. Patients were more explicit about the advantages and disadvantages that had played a role in their decision. They now knew what it meant to receive chemotherapy and they knew that, in spite of therapy, the tumour could return. This, in combination with the disappointment and the desperation that the revelation of the recurring tumour had generated, made it difficult for them to face up to another course of therapy. This did not mean, however, that they doubted whether they should undergo more treatment. On the one hand the unequivocal confirmation of their optimism during first-line therapy and on the other hand the realization and fear of approaching death strengthened patients' resolve to continue treatment. The avoidance of 'anticipated decision regret' probably also played a role. It was difficult for them to retrospectively conclude that first-line chemotherapy had been useless.

During first and second-line chemotherapy none of the patients voluntarily stopped treatment. One patient stopped third-line therapy even though it was effective. As the disease progresses, the tumour becomes more resistant and more difficult to treat. The longer therapy continues the more often the specialist has to terminate it because he finds that the tumour continues to develop in spite of therapy. During the course of treatment, the recurrence of the tumour and the deterioration of the patient's physical condition increase his despondency as to the use of further treatment. Most patients and their relatives noted, shortly before the patient's death, that they did not want to pursue treatment at the cost of all else.

Some patients were so sick that they were not able to make a (well-considered) choice. In such cases the responsibility lay with the specialist and he was the one who decided to treat. Most of the patients were still (physically) in good condition and could make the choice themselves, and the specialist advised them to agree to therapy. In practice, patients who did not want therapy, or who wanted to terminate therapy even though it was successful, had to persuade the specialist. If a patient doubted then the specialist introduced a 'pause' so that the patient could 'reconsider' before making the final decision. It seemed as though specialists required a more thoroughly considered decision in the case of patients who refused or broke off treatment than for those who simply accepted.

Verheggen has pointed out that the way in which specialists inform their patients, influences what patients decide (Verheggen 1996: 123). From the literature we know that patients are always inclined to follow the advice of their doctors (Siminoff and Fetting 1991). The specialists in this study readily admitted that they influenced the patient's choice of therapy by the way in which they provided information. For doctors in the Netherlands, treating a patient with small-cell lung carcinoma is the normal course of action. This assumption of normality filters down to the patient through the discourse of the doctor. For specialists discuss the prognosis if the patient refuses therapy but are silent regarding the prognosis with treatment, which makes the non-treatment option sound all the more threatening. Moreover, the specialist offers nothing other than therapy; the alternative is described as 'doing nothing' or 'wait and see'. By presenting the situation in this way the patient gets the impression that the choice is one between dying and living. The patient feels obliged to agree to therapy because the alternative is death ('I'm standing with my back against the wall'). The patient is put under pressure, but the alternatives suggested by the specialist are not the real ones. The real choice for the patient is not whether he is going to die but how soon. It is understandable that in this situation patients follow the doctor's advice.

The patient's treatment decisions are not determined solely by what the specialist says, however. There are various other factors that play a role, such as the patient's urge to be treated and the emotional resistance to doing 'nothing'. 'Nothing' means *nothing medical*. There is still much that can be done non-medically, such as providing emotional support. Patients would probably still agree to treatment, even if the doctor did not present the option with such verve. Research by Brinkman and others has shown that in phase 1 trials, even when patients receive written confirmation that they can expect no therapeutic effect from the treatment, half of them still agree to participate (Brinkman-Woltjer et al. 1988). The patients in this study were not always interested in knowing what they had agreed to. This does not mean, however, that patients simply agree with whatever the doctor suggests, but rather that when they agree it is for reasons other than those considered important from legal and ethical perspectives, i.e. reasons based on medical information. Patients have their own good reasons for accepting therapy, such as not wanting to be difficult, wanting to reciprocate or simply hope ('you never know').

In choices about palliative treatment it is not only a question of whether the patient can cope physically, but whether it is worth it for him. The patients I studied often did not want to choose and shifted the responsibility to the specialist. When the latter accepts this responsibility – even reluctantly – then he or she also accepts a moral obligation. As soon as the specialist becomes involved in the non-medical aspects of the choice, he or she is no longer only a medico-technical authority but also a *moral authority*. This is acceptable, but only if the specialist is prepared to recognize all the factors that are relevant for the patient's choice. This means that the specialist needs to know more about the patient and his or her situation. I have shown that patients discover the course of their illness in their own time. Sometimes they can cope with medical reality and other times they cannot. One moment patients refuse all responsibility while the next they are able to cope and feel the need to take control.

I have been focusing on the specialist, but caring for the patient is not exclusively the specialist's responsibility. For the patient the ideal would be a 'care team' in which all those involved in the care of the patient would cooperate. Perhaps it would be better if the specialists limited themselves to the medico-technical aspects of treatment and left the other aspects – including communication and support in taking difficult decisions – to others. Here the care relationship offers a solution. After all, what is important here is that during care attention should also be devoted to the context, the process and dynamics of the illness, and the patient's capacity to cope. It is also important to accept that the patient is sometimes confused and that the care provider temporarily takes over responsibility, only to give it back when the patient is able to cope again. Care should always be inspired by respect.

Informed consent perspective and care perspective

In this chapter I have discussed communication and choice, but I have in fact been talking about 'informed consent'. I now want to turn my attention to the gap between the law, ethics and practice. I will contrast what I observed during my study with the (theoretical) assumptions of 'informed consent' – the independent, active, autonomous, rational individual who wants to know, and who weighs the various options before deciding (Verkerk 1994: 7–8). Verheggen (1996) defines informed consent as the decision process that is based on adequate and properly understood information that results in well-considered and voluntary acquiescence or refusal of treatment or participation in a clinical trial. Informed consent is meant to protect patients from doctors who make decisions that are against their interests. In the Netherlands the Law on Medical-Scientific Research with Human Subjects has covered informed consent for medical research since January 1999, while routine medical treatment is covered by the *Wet op de Geneeskundige Behandelings Overeenkomst* (WGBO). In the case of routine treatment, the doctor has to inform the patient about his illness, the results of examinations and tests, and possible treatments. The patient, for his part, has to give informed consent. The rules for patients participating in scientific research are stricter. Patients must be informed, and they must confirm their agreement, in writing. The WGBO applied to all the patients I studied. In addition, some of them also participated in clinical trials (Mr Dekker and Mr Wiersema).

The information provided by the doctor should enable patients to judge their condition so that they can make appropriate decisions relating treatment and life-style (Roscam Abbing 1993: 25). The assumption is that the patient can only make a well-informed decision and be aware of what he is agreeing to on the basis of adequate information (Hulst 1995: 10). The information provided relates to facts, possibilities and expectations. It is important for the patient to be aware of the nature and goal of the proposed action, the possible alternatives, the expected outcomes and possible consequences of treatment versus abstention, the prognosis of the illness and the chances of recovery (Roscam Abbing 1995: 25). The doctor's obligation to inform the patient is also covered in the disciplinary rules of the medical profession. Obviously, the doctor cannot tell the patient everything; the content and the amount of information provided are partly determined by what the doctor suspects the patient already knows and the latter's capacity to cope. The doctor has the obligation to check whether the patient has understood important information. The duty to inform is based on the assumption that the patient must be given information about the facts and options that a reasonable person may expect to receive under the circumstances (Roscam Abbing 1995). Civil law review of the WGBO is based on good faith, reasonableness and fairness (Roscam Abbing 1995). Informed consent is also meant to give the doctor–patient relationship a different character. For example, Hulst notes that the 'well-considered consent' not only entails that the patient understands what he is consenting to, but also emphasizes that the relationship between doctor and patient should be one of equality. According to Hulst, the emphasis on the well-considered aspect of consent tends to correct the unequal relationship of dependency that exists in reality between patient and care provider (Hulst 1995: 4).

The problem is that the patients in this study often did not want to know and they usually felt no need to be actively involved in decisions about their treatment. Another lacuna is that, according to the informed consent perspective, people are consistent and unequivocal, as reflected in the WGBO. In this law there are two legal exceptions that forbid the care provider to inform the patient. The first is when the patient makes it clear that he does not want to be informed. This leaves little room for nuances and the patient has to make it unequivocally and explicitly clear that he does not want to know. This is precisely what the seriously ill patients I studied could not and would not do. It is often difficult for the healthy to be unequivocal about what they do and do not want, and it would be useful to recognize this ambiguity. The second exception is when the information will have serious negative consequences for the patient (Roscam Abbing 1995: 26–7), for example due to the increased risk of suicide (Hulst 1995).

The gap between rule and practice raises the obvious question of the value of legislation. My initial judgement was negative,[21] but I have since revised this. It is unavoidable that laws are highly abstract and based on the model citizen, and criticism on this level is easily given. Legemate has correctly pointed out that the relationship between law and reality is not 'bilateral'. There are various factors which, either alone or in combination, result in a discrepancy between rule and reality: poor communication, fear,

---

21 I adopted this point of view in my previous book (The 1997a).

powerlessness, lack of expertise or skills, disinterest, language problems, and lack of time. Many of these problems can be solved without calling the legitimacy of the legal intervention into question or having to alter the law (Legemate 1994: 20, my translation). There are always discrepancies between theory and practice and there are all kinds of (legal) entities that do not really exist. The point is to achieve the right balance. Legemate notes that, on the one hand, we must avoid a situation in which reality unjustly dictates the rules, but on the other hand it is also undesirable that 'by creating the rule we artificially maintain a legal situation which does not do justice to the way in which patients, care providers and health care institutions cope with dilemmas and complex issues' (Legemate 1994). The WGBO is an example of an openly formulated law that gives doctors the freedom to shape informed consent on the basis of their own experience. Article 7:453 of the Dutch penal code ('the care of a good care provider') states that it is not only the WGBO that should be important in determining the doctor's actions, but also the norms, knowledge and experience of the medical profession. The combination of WGBO and 'the care of a good care provider' create circumstances conducive to the phased trajectory of information provision on the long-term perspective of the illness (Legemate 1995: 11–12). The first relevant question (before the medical exception and the 'right not to know') is: what is the best way of informing the patient, given the nature and course of the illness and the individual characteristics of the patient. In addition to being a code of behaviour, 'the care of a good care provider' is also a way of establishing links with other norms, such as those professional norms described in the social science literature. From this it follows that more is expected from doctors than medico-technical expertise; they also have to be able to communicate with the patient and collaborate with colleagues. The link to professional norms and social scientific literature does not imply, however, that the doctor can ignore patients' rights included in the WGBO on the basis of attitudes dominant in the medical profession. According to this law, doctors are obliged to inform patients about their illness, even if the prognosis is unfavourable. Disciplinary procedure has determined that doctors should not deviate from this even if they fear that this will adversely affect the healing process or are unsure of the (exact) prognosis (Hulst 1995: 21). Doctors may, as I have mentioned, decide on the way in which they provide the information, and it may sometimes be useful to inform the patient gradually (Hulst 1995: 26). Even when patients insist on their right not to know, doctors still need to be aware of the possible consequences of this for their patients. If patients are not informed about the poor prospects they may not have the time to make the necessary arrangements (Roscam Abbing 1995: 28), say goodbye and prepare themselves for the approaching end.

There are two approaches to informed consent and autonomy: abstract and substantial. The abstract approach is focused on the rules and emphasizes formalities. In the substantial approach, respect for autonomy and informed consent are interpreted as helping patients to become aware of what they want and then supporting them to achieve this. For patients who are seriously ill, like those in this study, this means that they must be allowed to be themselves and to complete their life in a way that is appropriate to them. Autonomy and informed consent mean being able to decide yourself and are inseparably connected to the right of self-determination. But more importantly, people have a right to give form to their lives based on their own experiences, desires and beliefs. Here I do not mean to say that all patients should be aware of their approaching end, and that this realization is a precondition for a good death. What I mean is that in order to give informed consent substance, it is important to study the context and place what is happening to the patient in a wider context. Informed consent and autonomy are not static concepts; they get their substance from practice. What I am arguing for is a (more) individual and flexible form of counselling and support for patients. People who have avoided confronting unpleasant truths all their lives should be allowed to continue to do this in the final stage of their lives. But patients who can and want to face up to their approaching death and who attach value to the process of closure, should be given the necessary time and opportunity, and they should be supported in this if need be.

According to the abstract approach, the doctor has done his duty when he has informed the patient and offered therapy. If the patient then shifts the responsibility back to the doctor, then there is nothing wrong from a legal or ethical point of view. Specialists in particular hold this interpretation of informed consent. The Law on Medical-Scientific Research with Human Subjects demands that, in order to take part in a trial, the patient has to sign a statement confirming that he has agreed to participate. I often heard doctors apologize as they asked patients for consent: 'According to the law we have to get your signature for this.' Over the specialist's shoulder I followed the notes he wrote in the patient's file, 'Discussed the treatment options extensively with the patient. After serious consideration the patient has decided to accept therapy.' The formal approach is also illustrated in Verheggen's research. He describes doctors' answers when they are asked what informed consent means, 'a fiction,' 'a legal or bureaucratic obstacle to proper care,' 'a signature on a consent form' (Verheggen 1996: 121). Many doctors feel that they have done all they can when the patient has signed and they have noted in the file that the patient has consented. Obviously, a patient's signature on a form or a doctor's notes in the file do not prove that the patient has really understood what they have been told and knows what they have agreed to (see also Roscam Abbing 1995: 30–1). This became clear in some of the discussions I later had with widows of patients who had participated in a clinical trial; they asked me whether their husbands had participated in a scientific study. They remembered that their husbands had had to sign something, but they were not sure what it was or what it was for.

It is clear that the emphasis on the patient's signature and the notes in the clinical file deviates from the intention of the law. Used in this way, it serves more to cover the doctor legally ('Of course I informed the patient; look, here is his signature') than to protect the patient. I was initially appalled by the limitations of the abstract approach. I felt that, with regard to informed consent, doctors got off too easily and I tended to view patients as victims. The way I saw it, doctors used the formalistic approach in order to get patients to do something, which had nothing to do with informed consent and the autonomy of the patient. After a while, however, I understood the doctors' position better and realized that their abstract view was a logical consequence of the emphasis that is placed on legal rules. I began to understand the patients' position and wondered how much they were really fooled by the abstract approach. What do patients really want? At the moment that they have to decide about treatment, the patients in this study could not know how their illness would develop nor understand the consequences of treatment, both of which are necessary to choose wisely. The independent, active, autonomous and unequivocal patient who makes rational decisions is, in this situation, at best an abstraction and possibly even a caricature. Patients want 'something' to be done and they want it done quickly, and doctors oblige them. The patient does not want to, or cannot, decide and the doctor knows this, so the patient signs and the doctor makes notes in the file and together they *pretend that the patient has decided*. In this way doctor and patient jointly accommodate the imposed ideal of the autonomous patient making his own decision. They use the legalistic framework to bridge the gap between the fiction of autonomous patient and reality. In this way both doctor and patient avoid the responsibility.

There are sound reasons for both the WGBO and the Law on Medical-Scientific Research with Human Subjects, such as the protection of patients and the improvement of doctor–patient communication. The WGBO is a good law in the sense that it provides for – and therefore respects – professional norms and practical realization. Those involved – the doctors and patients in this study – also have good reasons for using the law in the way they do. But does this mean that all is well? No, because all is not well. The problem is that there is no workable concept for the development of a mode of treatment in which the care needs of the patient are central. Moreover, it is rather simplistic to think that the law by itself could have this far-reaching effect. The patients in this study were often desperate and wanted to be helped; their needs and desires cannot merely be reduced to autonomy and informed consent. A different understanding and different criteria are needed. Social reality cannot easily be understood in terms of contractual rationality, impartiality and neutrality (Manschot 1997). What patients need is a form of care and a caring relationship that is not catered for by the law or the various schools of liberal ethics. Ideally patients and care providers should be 'partners' in a common care-undertaking, which does justice to the patients' authenticity, supports their autonomy and respects them as people. In the practice that I have observed there is much more need for a 'care perspective' than for an 'information perspective'. There is need for an approach which, in addition to respect for the patient's right to decide, also attends to care, dependency and vulnerability; in which the norm is process-oriented, the subject is situated and particular, and which has an appropriate vocabulary.

The ethics of care contains various elements that link up with this, and in what follows I present a few illustrative quotations. The 'ethics of care' is opposed to conventional ethical theories, and in particular to the incapability of a reductionist and mechanistic approach of expressing lived reality (Verkerk 1997). 'We have begun to realize,' according to Manschot, 'that there has hardly been any room, in the modern way of life, for the obvious fact that people are not only independent and able to cope, but also vulnerable and mortal, and more or less dependent on the care of others during various phases of their lives . . . An ethics of care should therefore start with the question of how facets relating to physical vulnerability and finiteness can be integrated in the pattern of life of the free and autonomous individual' (Manschot 1997: 99, my translation).

In a discussion that begins with a newspaper description of an ordinary scene in a nursing home psycho-geriatric ward, Sevenhuijsen writes that in the public debate, ethical questions surface mainly in terms of rights, duties and qualifications. The newspaper article in question was prompted by the case of 'Martha U,' the nurse who had admitted to having killed nine seriously demented geriatric patients. Sevenhuijsen remarks correctly that the reality of everyday health care is hardly visible in the public debate. 'They hardly mention the nurses and care providers, the demented women eating marshmallows, or the daily moral interactions in geriatric care. Their judgement of the killer nurse would be clear: punishable behaviour which, at best, might be mitigated by labelling it a result of *non compos mentis*' (Sevenhuijsen 1996: 14). The importance of everyday descriptions of what happens in health-care settings – such as the newspaper article used by Sevenhuijsen or the ethnography in this book – is that attention is focused on other considerations and (local) rationalities than in the public debate. This enables the reader to understand why things 'happen as they do' in practice and, in Sevenhuijsen's words, extends an invitation to 'judge with care'. The problem with 'judging with care,' however, not only lies with the domination of political categories in determining justice but also in the cognitive attitudes that are usually related to notions of justice. Public judgement is usually related to distance, neutrality, and the ability to rise above particular perspectives. The care-related virtues such as compassion, attention, empathy and eye for detail are opposed to this and described as belonging to another domain, that of interpersonal and private relationships. The modern ideal of citizenship expects citizens to cut loose dependencies and loyalties in order to make free and independent choices (Sevenhuijsen 1996: 14–16).

In short, existing moral vocabulary is inadequate. In the care perspective the moral subject is not understood as an abstract construct, according to Verkerk, but as a situated and particular subject (what is best for *this* patient in *this* particular situation?). 'Autonomy,' according to the sociologist Verbeek-Heida, 'is something that needs to be continually redefined in specific situations and based on the experience of everyday life. Independence and autonomy only have meaning in those specific situations. Being dependent on care in a certain area implies some consideration and reorganization of how you think of yourself in order to be able to achieve the kind of autonomy and independence suitable to the new situation' (Verbeek-Heida 1998).

In care ethics, moral problems are primarily understood in terms of responsibility that the individual has towards others. Verkerk refers to care as the involved answer to the vulnerability and needs of others (Verkerk 1997: 96). According to her, care not only requires intervention but may also entail doing nothing (i.e. not interfering) (Verkerk 1997: 100). In the care relationship it is important that the patient receives involved attention, and that the care providers really confront the patient with his choices; that the patient has the opportunity to express what he thinks is important and that care providers get to know the patient better.[22]

---

22 Generally speaking, the relationship that nurses and GPs have with their patients is closer to such a care relationship than that between specialists and patients.

The collusion

Optimism about recovery

When I examined the problem of 'unjustified optimism' among patients with small-cell lung cancer I discovered that this optimism tended to be localized in the 'treatment' and 'remission' phases of the illness trajectory. Subsequent analysis confirmed my initial hypothesis that patients' optimism was partly related to what doctors told patients (and what they did not tell them) and by the way in which they told them. I analysed doctor-patient interactions as consisting of two parallel, sometimes conflicting, streams of information or patterns of communication, which I distinguished in two ways. First, there was information relating to the long-term and the short-term perspectives on the illness and, second, there were the domains of public and hidden information. I also made an attempt to unravel the ambiguities of the treatment context.

I have noted the homogenous character of what I found in different patients, especially in the early phases of the illness. After they had experienced a recurrence there was more variation between patients. In some patients there was a clearly developing realization of approaching death. Others maintained their optimism, though often against their own better judgement. It was clear that patients lived with different truths, and on the basis of these told different narratives. On closer scrutiny my initial analysis turned out to be incorrect: the optimism of patients during first-line therapy and remission was not unambiguous. The recovery narrative of patients in that phase is real. There are simultaneous feelings of desperation and uncertainty, however, but these are much less manifest, which is why I did not devote much attention to them in the early phases of the study.

When I looked for additional explanations of patients' optimism, apart from doctor-patient communication, I found that patients also learn to recite the socially propagated recovery narrative and that they live, as do we all, with different but simultaneous narratives. Through the different forms of communication and the diverse narratives, patients gradually develop an ambivalent realization of approaching death. Patients (and their loved ones) know what is happening, but at the same time they are unaware. Patients use this condition of 'knowing and not knowing' in their communication with others, and in this sense it is functional for them. I eventually discovered that the patient's power and influence over the communication process – and thus over the 'unjustified optimism' – was much greater than I had imagined possible.

The optimism about recovery stems to a large extent from a collusion between doctor and patient in which more attention is devoted to the long-term perspective compared to the short-term. Both parties are ambivalent. The doctor both does and does not want to inform the patient of the death sentence; the patient both does and does not want to hear it. Both are afraid of the confrontation with the medical truth and with each other. In their communication each has the other in a 'hold': the doctor wants to 'spare', the patient wants to be 'spared'. In this way the doctor avoids informing the patient about the long-term perspective and escapes into the details of the short-term perspective. For their part patients do not ask questions and do not force doctors to provide information about the final stages of their illness. As a result of this collusion the wider picture of the illness – that it almost certainly recurs in the short term and is fatal – is only made clear in its final stages. In this way both doctor and patient collaborate in a way that is understandable at the time but regretted by patients and loved ones retrospectively. On the one hand, optimism gives both patients and their relatives the strength to persevere and cope with the situation. On the other hand, the realization that this is an illusion is experienced as painful, and the acceptance of approaching death and the saying of goodbyes are constrained by the sudden realization that time is limited.

Model

This study has generated a model which helps to explain patients' optimism and facilitate the study of their need for care and information. In addition to the influence of personal biography and individual circumstance, there are a number of factors that contribute to a common pattern that applies to this group of small-cell lung cancer patients as a whole. First, the specific aetiology of small-cell lung cancer means that it affects a relatively homogeneous group: usually older, less educated men who have smoked heavily and who have COPD (chronic obstructive pulmonary disease). Second, the clinical trajectory of the illness is almost identical for all patients. Third, the medical approach to the illness is highly routine, even to the extent of being guided by protocols, as a result of which patients have almost identical experiences with the medical system. Fourth, patients get to know each other during treatment and as a result develop shared attitudes and expectations. As a result the entire patient population in the hospital, and not only those with lung cancer, is to a large extent socially homogenous.

As a result of these factors patients experience a common illness trajectory, from disbelief and denial to unjustified optimism (from the medical perspective) during treatment and, finally, acceptance of the unavoidable end. These five factors (the epidemiological characteristics of the patients, the specific characteristics of the illness itself, the type of treatment offered, cohort formation and regional culture) together offer an explanatory model for the homogenous illness trajectory as described in this study.

The question that now arises is whether this 'unjustified optimism' occurs in other patients. The optimism is dependent to a large extent on the extraordinary sensitivity of small-cell lung cancer to (first-line) chemotherapy. Optimism about recovery therefore seems less likely in the case of cancers that are less responsive to treatment. Moreover, the optimism is related to the practice of recommending treatment to all patients. In a later study of the response shift in quality of life measurements among patients with small-cell lung cancer, it became clear that in non-academic hospitals there was less pressure to undergo (second-line) treatment. When the choice of whether or not to accept treatment is more open, it appears that more information is provided about the advantages and disadvantages of therapy, and the goal of treatment (extending life) is made more explicit. It should be noted, however, that there is more pressure to treat in academic hospitals because the patients who go to such hospitals are more treatment oriented and there is a need to recruit patients into clinical trials. It is therefore possible that the optimism described in this book is related to the methods and culture of academic hospitals. Finally, it should be noted that, in reactions to the publication of results from this study in the *British Medical Journal* and the *Western Journal of Medicine*, doctors and patients claimed that the unjustified optimism I described and the causal mechanisms I suggested occur widely in the US and the UK in relation to various kinds of cancer (Iwashyna and Christakis 2001).

Patients' needs

One of the most striking things in this study was the limited time patients had left at the time they received their diagnosis. This time is valuable, and important for achieving closure. In addition to leave-taking and arranging financial matters, patients can develop, mature and grow spiritually in this relatively short time span. However, in the patients I followed, this time was dominated by hospital visits, despair, fear, medically unjustified optimism and increasing dependence on the health-care sector. I have seen how patients and their partners changed their lifestyle when they realized that all the treatment does is give an extension of life. They seemed to accept their fate more easily, not focus as rigidly on the future. They seemed more able to live in and enjoy the present, without cherishing false hope. I am not claiming that all patients responded in this way; I also saw patients, paralysed by the thought that they were going to die because the cancer continued to grow, just sitting in their chair and waiting for the end. I also saw patients on their deathbed, fighting to the bitter end.

Later, relatives told me that an appropriate dose of information on the long-term perspective, repeated at appropriate moments, might have led to a more conscious leave-taking, and might also have helped the process of mourning. It was felt that if there had been more discussion of the approaching end in the hospital then there was a greater chance that this would have got through to the patient, who would have had more chance to get used to the idea of death, with all the consequences of that realization. (These are the remarks of relatives reflecting on what happened and should be interpreted in that context.) They felt that imposing information was not the solution. People who are used to repressing unpleasant thoughts should not be forced to change at this late stage. 'My husband was never a talker,' one widow told me, 'so he certainly didn't start at the end'. This has consequences for the care providers' obligation to inform the patient as thoroughly as possible. In practice it is difficult to determine what patients want, whether they can cope and what the right moment is to inform them. Awareness of death is not necessarily the best option for everyone. Not knowing can also play a positive role. The collusion between doctor and patient did not arise for nothing, after all. The need for information and whether or not patients absorb this information depends on the situation and the phase of the illness in which the patient finds himself or herself. Doctors have not discharged their obligation to inform patients by merely applying the rules ('I told him, so it's not my fault if he doesn't know'), but only when the right moments have been carefully chosen and explored in dialogue with the patient. This cannot be formalized in protocols, but must proceed by finding out how aware the patient is and adjusting the provision of information accordingly. A phased, repeated and individually adjusted process seems the proper way of providing patients with information about the long-term perspective of their illness. What I mean is that the patient's experience of the final phase of life is determined by those who provide the palliative and life-extending treatment. By treating, care providers interfere with the patient's life – by making choices and raising expectations that are closely related to what they think is good for the patient – and as a result it is not only medical-technical factors that play a role in this group of patients. This is another reason why it is inadequate to discuss only the short-term perspective with small-cell lung cancer patients.

Patients like the ones in this study cannot be treated 'normally,' and that is something that is insufficiently realized. Those who treat these patients also have a responsibility for providing psychosocial support and for channelling the gradually developing awareness of the outcome of the illness. Almost all patients said they would have liked to have received more time and attention. Mr Wiersema poignantly expressed the desire of most patients when he said he would like to phone the doctor in the evening and go over everything again. In the evening the stress of full waiting rooms and insistent pagers would be absent. In the evenings Mr Wiersema became aware of all the things he had not quite grasped, he remembered the questions he had meant to ask and he had more courage to discuss difficult topics.

Many patients expressed a need for more psychosocial support. They wanted more attention to be devoted to the personal consequences and the meaning of their illness in their daily lives. There were all kinds of practical problems: 'How are we going to tell the children?', 'How should I take care of my dying husband?', 'What should I be keeping an eye on?', 'What about those who remain behind?'. Every patient seemed to have an important 'secret' that had to be 'confessed' and sorted out before they died: a child who had broken off contact, a problematic marriage, or the death of a loved one. And of course there was a need for reflection on basic questions about the meaning of things. I found it striking that patients and their relatives often told me that they valued my 'listening ear'. The doctors and nurses were often too busy, patients did not like to 'impose on' relatives, and such matters were often too confrontational for friends. These discussions were not always about 'serious' topics, but often about everyday matters.

Another problem is that treatment consists of a large number of smaller parts. From a medical perspective this need not be a problem. Of course there are gaps, but generally treatment is good and what one care provider has done is reported to others involved with the same patient. Psychosocial support is more problematic. All those involved with the patient contribute to some extent, but none is aware of what others have done and there is certainly no coordination. If there is any handover then it is usually inadequate. In the outpatient clinic and on the wards patients are involved with numerous doctors and nurses. It would improve patient care if all these different elements in the treatment process were unified by establishing a system of medical and psychosocial coordination.

Avoiding responsibility

The above summary of patients' needs is rather obvious. The real question is why these have not been met. One important barrier is that due to lack of time, the routine nature of much clinical practice, other priorities, and interpretations of their role, doctors are not inclined to invest time and energy in understanding the details of patients' choices. They want to avoid emotional confrontations. Nurses think that it is the doctor's job to inform patients. Doctors think that psychosocial support should be left to the nurses and the patient's GP. Patients just want to get better, and they put all their trust in the doctors.

During the illness trajectory of patients with small-cell lung cancer all participants seem to hide. There are problems that are visible to all but which no one can solve and the alibi is always 'the organization of the hospital'. Everyone claimed to feel responsible, but in practice this responsibility was placed elsewhere. Problems were defined as someone else's, or at least as not being 'part of my job'. Everyone served 'the process' but no one stopped to question it. They preferred to concentrate on short-term tasks and thus avoid confronting the long-term issues. It often seemed to me like a group of people, each one trying to repair part of an old bicycle, without anyone considering whether it would ever be used again. I experienced this limited, almost parochial responsibility most strongly while studying end-of-life decisions on the intensive care (IC) ward. Patients were regularly fixed up so that they were well enough to be discharged from IC; what would happen to them after that, and whether or not that was desirable, was hardly mentioned. It was as though no one thought any further than the swinging doors of the IC ward; the inevitable problems that would arise on the other side were not considered. That was not part of the IC staff's (formal) responsibility. In this fragmented situation there is a shortage of 'long-term thinkers' who can keep an eye on the red thread and guide patients through the illness trajectory. I am not arguing against hospital specialists, but against the 'speeding train' in which they are all sitting, and in which the lack of honesty – or rather fear of honesty – is so striking. The moral responsibility that I ascribe to the specialists does not rest on each of them personally; it is the responsibility of the whole team caring for the patient. If the specialist does not have the time or feels that he or she is not the right person to provide this aspect of care, then someone else in the team could do it. The point is that someone in the team needs to take responsibility for directing the meeting of the patient's needs.

This responsible person would need to follow the patient with small-cell lung cancer (and his or her relatives) through the illness trajectory, both in the hospital and at home. At present, as far as I am aware, care providers operate either inside the hospital or outside, and if they do have contact with each other it is only sporadic. The moment at which the hospital decides that nothing more can be done is painful for patients because it signals a break in contact with the hospital. Specialists insist that patients are still welcome, but in practice it means that hospital visits do diminish at the very least and a new phase in the illness is initiated in which the GP is central. What I have learnt from this study is that illness trajectories are dynamic wholes that consist of different but related phases. When I asked patients who I met in the hospital but who were not participants in my study about their illness, they proceeded chronologically, starting their stories at the moment when they noticed the first symptoms. To understand it is important to see the whole and not the smaller parts. The 'responsible person' I am suggesting should be part of the care offered by the hospital and there to bridge obstacles to the continuity of care and psychosocial support. This is no easy task. The relationship with patients and their relatives should not be one of opposing parties but rather a kind of long-term care relationship. In addition to expertise, such a relationship also requires courage, time and, especially, motivation. This role will have to form the pivot of the relationship between the different parties.

Care director

I have given a lot of thought to the question of who should take on this role. One possibility is someone trained in the provision of psychosocial care, such as a clinical psychologist or a social worker. (It is striking that there were many such people in the Ruysdael Clinic, but I seldom saw them on the wards where there was such a need for psychosocial care.) A disadvantage of this, however, is that it would add an additional person to the many already involved in the treatment and care of these patients. My preference is therefore for someone who is already involved. One option is the specialist. The most important disadvantage of this has already been mentioned: specialists do not want to play this role. There are also good arguments for choosing someone other than the person with medical responsibility. Moreover, my study has shown that the specialist and the patient collude. This means that this relationship can only be broken open by introducing a third party, someone who can intervene in the bad news interview when the discussion turns to treatment and say, 'We're not going to decide on that now. I'll discuss everything with the family, then they can discuss it among themselves, and only then are we going to make a decision'. The GP could play this role. Ideally, the GP has the advantage of having known the patient before the illness and can make a more balanced judgement about the patient's situation. Moreover, the patient is usually discharged from the hospital and into the care of the GP for the final, terminal phase of the illness. GPs also generally have more of an eye for the non-medical aspects of the illness and they are often more reflective and critical about treatment than the hospital specialists. In the context of a fellowship that I received from the Netherlands Cancer Society (Nederlandse Kander Bestrijding), I interviewed GPs about this option and they confirmed my impression. But there are barriers to GPs taking on this role. The patients in my study came from towns and villages far from the Ruysdael Clinic, making regular hospital visits by the GP impracticable. There were also barriers relating to medical insurance, and some GPs did not want an extra psychosocial responsibility, partly because this was seen as being a 'leftover' from the hospital. These interviews were relatively superficial and it would be useful to study further the mutual tensions between hospital specialists and GPs in relation to life-extending and palliative care.

The final option, appointing a nurse as care director, seems to be the best, and in the Ruysdael Clinic the best candidates would be the oncology nurses in the outpatient clinic. There are a number of reasons for this preference. Nurses are involved in the care of the patient in both a medical and a psychosocial role. They are accessible to patients and the relationship is less tense than that between patients and psychologists, for example. Because of their position, nurses are able to understand all the parties and as a result can negotiate, mediate and guide. They are part of the hospital care system and are familiar with its culture, dominant discourse and codes of behaviour. The nurse as care director would have to ensure continuity. He or she would need to be present during the important consultations between specialist and patient in the outpatient clinic, visit the patient on the ward, maintain contact with the junior ward doctors, and be present when the patient is discussed. In addition he or she would also have to act as a care provider. I am aware that a care director would not provide a solution to all the problems and gaps in care that I have enumerated. It is an attempt to address a need expressed by those confronted by these problems in practice. If such a role was created, this would not excuse us from continuing to think about better solutions.

Self-care

Another factor that should receive attention is the discourse. In the dominant medical culture 'the solution' and curing the illness are primary. The meaning of all this for the patient and his or her life comes after this. The patients I studied did not get better. Indeed, they all died relatively quickly. From a medical point of view there is not much to say. Patients have to learn to live with the reality. This requires a language that is not merely medical, a language in which emotions, intuition and doubt have a role. The question, 'can this illness be cured?' should be related to the question, 'what is the meaning of this confrontation with vulnerability for the patient and how does he or she want to deal with this in everyday life?'. Here it is not recovery from the illness that should be central but the working through of what is to come.

And this brings me to the responsibility of the patient for caring for himself or herself. We must take care not to fall into the trap of accepting the current vogue and assuming that the patient is a victim who must be taken care of. If people are responsible for their own lives, then surely they are still responsible when they are ill, old, lonely and dying? There is silence, according to the philosopher Verkerk (2000), about what Socrates called 'taking care of yourself'. This care requires self-knowledge or self-understanding: who am I, what do I want, and what is important for me in this life? It also requires the development of an attitude towards various important aspects of life such as health, illness, death, old age, friendship, work and love. Self-care consists primarily in continually ascribing meaning to one's own existence, especially when this is affected by radical changes. The task is to relate to changed circumstances: how do I ascribe meaning to my life now that it has changed so radically? This requires that from an early age people think about how they want to give form to their lives, how they relate to life, and what they consider important. People must learn to be flexible and how to cope with vulnerability and mortality. By taking responsibility for his or her own life, the patient can become an active participant in the care process.

The fear of failure, one of the great modern taboos, is identified by the sociologist and historian Richard Senett (2001) as the cause of this contemporary avoidance of responsibility. Admitting to failure, giving it form and a place in our biography is painful, and we do not discuss it with others. Perhaps we should learn that dependence, inequality, suffering, sickness and death are part of life, that life is not always pleasant, and that when it is not it is not up to others to establish a new equilibrium, but our own responsibility. Life can be hard work, and perhaps it would be good to focus more attention on this. We should see things more proportionately and have an ear not only for the success stories, but for all the other narratives as well. No matter how much we would wish it to be otherwise, in the struggle against disease and mortality, humankind is the weaker side. Society has to recognize the limits to medicine and correct the exaggerated expectations that have developed. We must learn to realize that suffering is part of life, that life cannot always be 'made,' and that death cannot be postponed (Dunning 1999). Having said that, I have to admit that I am not entirely sure what the best solution to this complex set of problems is. The role of care director and giving the patient more responsibility are two possible options, but they are not *the* solution.

Epilogue

Relatives reflect

As the train stops I wind down the window and survey the platform. I see Mrs Wiersema, holding a cake in a white cardboard box, scanning the train. I observe her for a moment before attracting her attention. She has not changed.

'Mrs Wiersema, I'm over here,' I call, waving. She smiles and walks to the nearest door. We embrace in the corridor. We immediately fall into a conversation about the subject that binds us: the period that we were both linked, for such very different reasons, to the Ruysdael Clinic. Half an hour later the train stops and we step down onto the platform where Johan, Vera and Roosje are waiting for us. The five of us drive to Mrs Dekker's house. The last time I was there, Mr Dekker lay in the living room in his coffin. We talk about our shared time in the hospital. Three years have passed, but the events are as vivid as though they had happened yesterday: the early days with the moods of euphoria on the ward, Mr Wiersema dancing round the room, the jokes about crates of beer on the balcony. But also the pain, the sickness, the fear and the sadness. We talk about the waiting room and its population of fellow-sufferers, the Kosters, the nervous Mr Bokjes, and about Dr Liem, Dr Veerman and Dr Heller. We talk about everything and everybody. Finally I ask Mrs Wiersema and Mrs Dekker whether, with hindsight, they would have done anything differently.

'Were Klaas and Joop participating in research?' Mrs Dekker asks. I nod. 'Klaas thought that the needles were the worst,' she says. At the end he couldn't cope with that any more. If we could do it all over again, I'd try and persuade him not to participate in the research. I'm not sure whether I'd succeed, though. Klaas agreed to everything. He didn't like to complain and be difficult. He thought it was terrible when I questioned what was going on. He'd say that we needed to trust them. He surrendered himself completely to the doctors.

'You were always there,' Mrs Wiersema says. 'When we talk about those days we always mention you. Remember the last time he was admitted?' I nod. 'He always hated it when they admitted him. I came during visiting hours and who was already there on the edge of the bed? You.' She wipes her eyes. 'Child, you still remember everything, and you had to deal with so many patients.'

'There were other patients,' I say, 'but you were always special. You were the first and that's different. It's something I can't forget.'

'You must know much more than we do,' Mrs Dekker says. 'You spent so many hours talking to them. You were with them in the hospital when we were at home. They probably told you things they never told us.'

I know that I had waited too long before getting in touch. After the funerals we had exchanged the odd card and phone call. I kept promising to visit but never quite got round to it. I have the feeling that I abandoned them at a time when they needed support. I wonder how I should have acted; whether there are rules for that sort of thing. It is good that we are together now, though. It is good to talk about past experiences. But this is also a parting, and we all know it. Our lives are too different to continue sharing them. We have had an intensive experience together but the episode is in need of closure.

'The most difficult thing is that we never discussed his death,' Mrs Wiersema is saying. 'If I could do things over then that's something I'd do differently. He knew that he was dying. You feel something like that coming. But he just wasn't the type to talk about it. So we never discussed it.'

'Klaas felt that he was going to die, and he was ready for it,' Mrs Dekker says. She is still happy that they had been able to say goodbye in full awareness. She thinks it was good for him as well. 'He was always a step ahead of us in the process of coming to terms with the fact that he was dying. That's why he had to go through the process alone. He had already come to terms with it when the time came to die, whereas we still had to start.'

'It would have been better for us if we had talked about it,' Mrs Wiersema says. 'Especially when I hear how you went about things. It's a pity it didn't work out like that for us.' Mrs Wiersema is not sure, however, whether it would have been better for her husband if they had discussed things. 'He was never a talker,' she says, shrugging.

Mrs Wiersema is also troubled by the fact that her son regrets not having been there during that last Christmas. If he'd realized that it was the last Christmas then he would have been there. 'Maybe the doctors should have been more clear about the fact that it was the end,' she says. 'I never heard them say that clearly. If they'd have done so it might have got through to us how serious the situation really was. But as it was, we kept on hoping. The X-rays were clear and we thought that things were going to be okay. Maybe we would have talked if it wasn't for the hope. Maybe if they'd been clearer we wouldn't have had so much hope.'

'But you need that hope to continue fighting,' Mrs Dekker says. She is not sure whether the doctors should have been clearer.

'Yes but when someone says you're not going to get better, you don't immediately think you're going to die,' Mrs Wiersema says.

Mrs Dekker thinks it is important how things are presented. She found the conversation with Dr Racz very useful; it had been the breakthrough that finally led to her understanding the nature of the illness.

'I think that if I were 70 and I had cancer, I wouldn't accept treatment,' Mrs Wiersema says suddenly. 'All those side effects. No, that's not for me. Maybe . . . maybe I would even refuse treatment if I had it now.'

Mrs Dekker can understand, but she does not agree. Her life has regained some of its colour, especially since the birth of her granddaughter. Now there are things that are worth living for again.

Both women say that at the time they needed more time and attention from the doctors. Everything was new and strange and they had so many questions. They would have appreciated a meeting with the doctor afterwards as well, so that he could explain things. Mrs Dekker had phoned Dr Liem after her husband's funeral. She was determined to ask him all the questions that were troubling her, but when it came to the crunch the questions dried up. Dr Liem did not offer much information either. 'Everything comes at you and you feel such a need to talk. That's why it was so nice that you were there,' she says, looking at me. 'You can't talk to your relatives like that; you don't want to burden them. You listened to us and that was enough.'

'It would be a good idea to have someone like you in the hospital,' Mrs Wiersema says. 'Someone who knows what's happening, who's been to all the meetings and who gives you attention.'

The role, influence and dilemmas of the researcher

Just as in everyday life, I did not have the same relationships with all the participants in my study. I got on well with some patients and their relatives and less so with others. With some I discussed existential matters relating to their illness, with others I joked, trying to cheer them up, and with yet others I listened to interminable stories of children, grandchildren and football. It was impossible not to be more involved with some than with others. And later, when they died, I noticed that the deaths of some affected me more than those of others (Cannon 1989: 72).

It happened gradually. At first it was only the odd incident and I hardly noticed what was happening. Later I had to admit to myself that sheer neutral observation was not possible. As time went by I acquired a role. Informants had already started asking me questions in an early stage of the study: about their medical situation, about what exactly the doctor had said during a consultation, and about what I thought they should do. I received an increasing number of phone calls at home, especially during the weekends, from worried partners of patients. Then one day in the hospital

I received a direct appeal. It started with Mrs Dekker paging me through Dr Liem during an outpatient consultation in order to ask her big question, 'Have they given him up?' Following my suggestion she made an appointment to see the doctor. During that meeting she kept looking at me, imploring help, each time she asked a question. I kept nodding encouragingly. She cried, at first because of anger, later due to grief. Whether I liked it or not, I had become a player in what I was studying. Sometimes I was unwillingly absorbed into the process, and sometimes I had to counter my inclination to intervene. Like the time the Dekkers were arguing about whether to go on holiday this year or postpone it until next year. I had to make an effort not to shout, 'Do it now; there won't be a next year'. Simultaneously I also thought, 'Who am I to remain silent and deprive them of that last holiday together?' I said nothing. Two months later Mr Dekker had a recurrence and he died six months after the discussion about the holiday. When I think of the holiday that they will now never be able to have together, I still feel guilty.

In the beginning I switched effortlessly from one perspective to the other. In the outpatient clinic I spent an increasing amount of time sitting with patients in the waiting room, sharing their worries. But the time always came that I changed sides, taking my place next to the doctor and opposite those who had taken me into their confidence a few minutes earlier. Because the specialist briefed me before consultations, I always knew more about patients' illness than they did themselves. I always pretended that these role changes were quite normal, but actually they were confusing. 'Whose side am I really on?' was a question that I kept asking myself. One day, at the beginning of a consultation the doctor was still busy sorting his papers. On the opposite side of the table Mr Wiersema made eye contact with me and raised his eyebrows questioningly, gesturing with his head toward the latest X-rays hanging on the light box. Before I realized what I was doing I was nodding reassuringly. Mr Wiersema nudged his wife and they both sighed, relieved. I had been sucked into the drama without being able to anticipate the consequences.

Later I realized that the ease with which I nodded was based partly on the fact that at the time Mr Wiersema's medical situation was favourable. But by nodding I had manoeuvred myself into an impossible position. The day would come when Mr Wiersema would look at me questioningly from across the table and I would not be able to nod reassuringly. 'You must be more alert,' I told myself. 'It's the doctor who should be giving the information, not you'. But was it possible to abstain? Could I pretend to know nothing when Mr Wiersema was appealing to me for information?

A short while later I noticed that it was not only my explicit behaviour that conveyed information. During a discussion with a patient and his partner, shortly before the latter's death, I realized that I was emitting implicit signals as well. We were discussing the morning on which they had been told that the chemotherapy was not working and that the CT-scan had revealed metastases. Suddenly the partner said, 'We knew before the doctor told us. We saw it in the way you greeted us. Roel said, "Her face says everything; things are not good" '. At that moment I realized that however hard I tried to be neutral, I was still going to influence the object of my study.

Occasionally I worried that I was a burden on the patients and their relatives. I did not want to make an already stressful situation worse. Even though I had received ethical clearance for the study, I wondered whether what I was doing was really ethically acceptable. On the other hand I noticed that I provided support that was appreciated. I was always there, I had time, I listened, I was interested. I struggled with this dilemma for a while, but I am now convinced that my contribution was a positive one. Patients and their partners told me this often. Some thought that there should be 'someone like me' in the hospital permanently. After the death of a patient I often received messages from relatives saying that they had found the contact with me pleasant. Doctors and nurses confirmed that patients had been positive about my involvement.

Even though I provided support to patients and their relatives, I still 'used' them. I did not only listen to them with a sympathetic ear, I listened and observed as a researcher. This still sometimes made me uneasy. Another problem was ending the relationship with relatives after the patient had died. The job was done, but the affection that had developed through the sharing of intimate moments was still there. I visited the bereaved families at home and I attended most funerals. But then, perhaps when the bereaved families needed most support, I distanced myself. This sometimes clashed with what I felt I should be doing, but it was practically impossible for me to maintain contact.

Between detachment and involvement

Much has been written about the practice of ethnographic research. Often hidden in the appendices of ethnographies are the stories of gaining access, language barriers, cultural misunderstandings, and details of the research process. There is usually little discussion of the dilemmas and the emotional pain (Shaffir et al. 1980: 3–4). In this epilogue I attempt to make the emotional aspects of fieldwork visible. I have shown how the contact with informants was established and how it developed during the course of the research. The book is a personal narrative of encounters and a description of situations in which I participated. But it also gives an impression of my attempts not to disturb what I was studying; it shows how I struggled to achieve the proper balance between involvement and detachment. In what follows I will discuss the problems of emotional involvement and the implications of this for the results and presentation of the study.

Ethnographers develop extensive relationships of trust with their informants and through these they collect their information. But these relationships also put them in a dilemma. Ethnographers are told that emotional involvement impedes objective scientific study. As Pool has pointed out, 'In the social sciences, writing about the emotional involvement of the researcher is generally considered taboo, and in anthropology any discussion of personal involvement is often relegated to what is contemptuously described as confession ethnography' (Pool 2000: 10). On the other hand, however, ethnographers are told that some attachment to informants is necessary for understanding (Katz Rothman 1986: 46). If you try to maintain objective distance, you miss the experiential aspects of the lives of those you are studying. But this also has its attractive side; it means you do not have to experience certain stressful or unpleasant situations such as the death of an informant to whom you are particularly attached (Oakley 1986: 252). I am now convinced that emotional involvement is part of every relationship of trust, whether or not it is private or work-related. It is perhaps exaggerated to claim that the involvement of a researcher with an informant goes as deep as personal relationships, but there is certainly emotional involvement.

The relationship of trust between researcher and informant is necessary, but not without consequences for the researcher (Oakley 1986: 248). I was moved when I stood with Mrs Dekker in front of her husband's coffin in the living room. It was not simply 'a tragic situation' for her; I really felt miserable. When I sat at the bedside of the dying Mr Wiersema, it was not just the death of an arbitrary patient. I saw vividly before me our meetings in the waiting room, the consultations, the stays on the ward. I saw Mr Wiersema waving to me in the rain, on the hospital parking lot; I saw him whispering to *Sinterklaas* and the *Zwarte Piet* giving me a handful of ginger biscuits. I remembered that morning on the ward, the morning of the failed resuscitation, when Mr Wiersema's door had been closed. It had become impossible for me to see Mr Wiersema and Mr Dekker as merely objects of study (Smith Bowen 1956: 163).

It would be going too far to say that this study altered my life, but it did affect me. I now see the health-care sector, illness and death differently. More importantly perhaps, is the insight it has given me about myself as researcher. In this sense my informants were participants in the process of my own development. I was already aware that ethnographers are supposed to be their own research instruments. During this study I experienced that this instrument is human and not a neutral machine. I learned that there is a continuum between two poles, involvement and detachment, and that the relationship between researcher and informant is dynamic and moves continually between these poles.

My most important discovery was that the human aspects of the ethnographer-as-research-instrument – those aspects that I initially tried to suppress – are not a weakness but a strength. Because I was emotionally involved it was easier to empathize and to understand (to an extent) what it means to be terminally ill, to have a loved one who is dying, to lose someone dear to you. It was also easier to understand those who treat and care for the terminally ill. I know from my own experience that this is much more difficult with a more detached attitude and when using more detached methods such as questionnaires. The most important difference between these two methods is that being involved does not only generate data, but also emotions, insight and experience. I now understand how patients and their relatives repress bad news because I have done so myself. Mr Dekker's death took me completely by surprise, even though I knew they could do nothing more for him and was aware that he had said goodbye to me in the outpatient clinic. I did not want him to die and so I did not see that he was dying. I now also understand how difficult it is for doctors to deal with dying patients; how difficult it is to determine how far their awareness of approaching death has developed. I know from my own experience how important it is to have that small glimmer of hope in the darkness of despair.

Finally, the researcher has to pass on this knowledge and understanding to the reader. The process of development that I experienced can also benefit others. I became wiser because I was prepared to open myself up emotionally. My emotional involvement also had an effect on the way in which I can present my story: by describing my own emotional experience I wanted to evoke emotions in the reader. In this way I hoped to increase understanding of terminal illness and the emotional aspects that are so essential. I know now that using a distanced approach, I would not have learned what I have learned through involvement. I know that it is only through involvement that I could tell my story in such a way that my patients would really live.

Bibliography

Anonymous (1984) Consent, how informed? *The Lancet*, 331: 1445–7.

Anonymous (1991) Consent, how informed? *The Lancet*, 338: 665–6.

Anspach, R.R. (1993) *Deciding Who Lives. Fateful Choices in the Intensive-Care Nursery*. Berkely, CA: University of California.

Applebaum, P. (1988) Assessing patients capacities to consent to treatment, *New England Journal of Medicine*, 319: 165–8.

Aries, P. (1981) *The Hour of Our Death*. London: Allen Lane.

Armstrong, D. (1984) The patients view, *Social Science and Medicine*, 18: 7437–44.

Armstrong, D. (1987) Silence and truth in death and dying, *Social Science and Medicine*, 24: 651–7.

Bensing, J. (1991) Doctor–patient communication and the quality of care, *Social Science and Medicine*, 32: 1301–10.

Bignold, S., Ball, S. and Cribb, A. (1994) *Nursing Families with Children with Cancer: The Work of the Paedietric Oncology Outreach Nurse Specialists*. A report to Cancer Relief Macmillan Fund and the Department of Health.

Bolt, I. (1991) *Informed consent: De patiënt wikt, de arts beschikt? Een verkennend theoretisch en empirisch onderzoek*. Amsterdam: Vrije Universiteit.

Brinkman-Woltjer, L.F.J., Vermorken, J.B., van Groeningen, C.J., Gall, H.E. and Pinedo, H.M. (1988) Fase 1-onderzoek als niet-therapeutisch experiment in de oncologie, *Nederlands Tijdschrift Voor Geneeskunde*, 132(51): 2321–5.

Britten, N. (1991) Hospital consulant's views of their patients, *Sociology of Health and Illness*, 13(1): 83–94.

Buunk, B.P., Collins, R.L., Taylor, S.E., van Yperend, N.W. and Dakof, G.A. (1990) The affective consequences of social comparison: either direction has its ups and downs, *Journal of Personal and Social Psychology*, 59: 1138–49.

Cannon, S. (1989) Social research in stressful settings: difficulties for the sociologist studying the treatment of breastcancer, *Sociology of Health and Illness*, 11: 62–77.

Casselith, B.R., Zupkis, R., Sutton-Smith, K. et al. (1980) Informed consent – Why are its goals imperfectly realized? *The New England Journal of Medicine*, 302: 16.

Costain Schou, K. (1993) Awareness contexts and the construction of dying in the cancer treatment setting: 'micro' and 'macro' levels in narrative analysis, in L. Clark (ed.) *The Sociology of Death*. Oxford: Blackwell Publishers, 238–63.

Costain Schou, K. and Hewison, J. (1999) *Experiencing Cancer: Quality of Life in Treatment*. Buckingham: Open University Press.

Coulton, C. (1990) Decision making in support: patient perceptions and preference, *Journal of Clinical Epidemiology (suppl.)*, 43: 51s–54s.

de Swaan, A. (1985) *Het medisch regiem*. Amsterdam: Meulenhoff.

Degner, L.F. and Sloan, J.A. (1992) Decision making during serious illness: what role do patients really want to play? *Journal of Clinical Epidemiology*, 45(9): 941–50.

Dunning, A.J. (1999) Betoverde wereld; over ziek en gezond in onze tijd. Amsterdam: Meulenhoff.

Dupuis, H.M. (1988) *Schijn en werkelijkheid*, onder red. van D.P. (et al.) Boerhave Commissie, Leiden.

Elias, N. (1990) *De eenzaamheid van stervenden in onze tijd*. Amsterdam: Meulenhoff.

Ende J., Kazis, L., Ash, A. et al. (1989) Measuring patients' desire for autonomy; decision making and information-seeking preferences among medical patients, *Journal of General Internal Medicine*, 4: 23–30.

Faden, R.R. and Beauchamp, T.L. (1986) *History and Theory of Informed Consent*. New York/Oxford: Oxford University Press.

Fallowfield, L. (1993) Giving sad and bad news, *The Lancet*, 341: 476–8.

Fallowfield, L.J., Baum, M. and Maguire, P. (1986) Effect of breast conservation on psychological morbidity associated with diagnosis and treatment of early breast cancer, *British Medical Journal*, 293: 1331–4.

Faulkner, A., Argent, J., Jones, A. and O'Keeffe, C.O. (1995) Improving the skills of doctors in giving distressing information, *Medical Education*, 29: 303–7.

Finch, J. and Wallis, L. (1993) Death, inheritance and the lifecourse, in L. Clark (ed.) *The Sociology of Death*. Oxford: Blackwell Publishers, pp. 50–68.

Fontaine, B., Kloos, P. and Schrijvers, J. (1990) Theoretische vernieuwing en de betekenis van feministische antropologie, in B. Fontaine, P. Kloos and J. Schrijvers (eds) *De crisis voorbij; persoonlijke visies op vernieuwing in de antropologie*. Leiden: DSWO Press Rijksuniversiteit.

Frank, A.W. (1995) *The Wounded Storyteller; Body, Illness, and Ethics*. Chicago, IL: The University of Chicago Press.

Gelauff, M. and Manschot, H. (1997) Zingeving als funderende dimensie van zorg; voorstel voor een perspectiefwisseling op de zorgrelatie, in: M. Verkerk (red.) *Denken over zorg; concepten en praktijken*. Utrecht: Elsevier/De Tijdstroom, 189–205.

Gilbar, O. (1989) The attitude of the doctor to the refusal of the cancer patient to accept chemotherapy, *Medicine and Law*, 8: 527–34.

Gilbert, N. (1993) *Researching Social Life*. London: Sage.

Glaser, B.G. and Strauss, A.L. (1965) *Awareness of Dying*. New York: Adline Publishing Company.

Groen, H.J.M., The, B.A.M., Sanderman, R., de Vries, E.G.E. and Mulder, N.H. (1995) Quality of life in lungcancer patients treated by radiation with and without carboplatin, in H.J.M. Groen (red.) *Exploration of New Therapy for Lung Cancer*, proefschrift, Rijksuniversiteit Groningen, pp. 95–105.

Hack, T.F., Degner, L.F. and Dyck, D.G. (1994) Relationship between preferences for decisional control and illness information among women with breast cancer: a quantitative and qualitative analysis, *Social Science and Medicine*, 39: 193–6.

Hak, T., ten Have, P. and Goethals, A. (1997) Kwalitatieve medische sociologie: nut en noodzaak, in A. Goethals, T. Hak and P. ten Have (ed.) *Kwalitatieve medische sociologie*. Amsterdam: SISWO, pp. 5–19.

Hammersley, M. and Atkinson, P. (1995) *Ethnography; Principles in Practice*. London: Routledge.

Henneman, E.A. (1995) Nurse-physician collaboration: a poststructuralist view, *Journal of Advanced Nursing*, 22: 359–63.

Howe, E. (ed.) (1994) Approaches (and possible contraindications) for enhancing patients' atonomy, *The Journal of Clinical Ethics*, 5: 179–88.

Hulst, E.H. (1995) *Het recht van de patient op informatie: de juridische stand van zaken*. Utrecht: KNMG (KNMG-Project 'Informed Consent').

Iwashyna, T.J. and Christakis, N.A. (2001) Physicians, patients, and prognosis (Commentary on: B.A.M. The, A. Hak, G.H. Koëter and G. van der Wal, Collusion in doctor-patient communication about imminent death: an ethnographic study.) *Western Journal of Medicine*, 174(4): 253–4.

Jansen, H. (1998) De boekenrubriek nieuwe stijl: auteurs schrijven terug, *Kwalon (Tijdschrift voor kwalitatief onderzoek in Nederland)*, 3(8): 40.

Kastelein, W.R. (1995) Informatieplicht en toestemmingsvereiste, *Medisch Contact*, 13: 336–41.

Kastelein, W.R. (1993) Arts, patiënt en recht: zelfbeschikking en recht op informatie, waar ligt de grens?, in R.J.M. Dillmann, E. van Leeuwen and G.K. Kimsma (eds) *Ethiek in de medische praktijk*. Utrecht: Bunge, pp. 60–70.

Katz Rothman, B. (1986) Reflections: On hard work, *Qualitative Sociology*, 9: 48–53.

Katz, J. (1984) *The Silent World of Doctor and Patient*. New York/London: Collier Macmillan Publishers.

Kellehear, A. (1992) *Dying of Cancer; The Final Year of Life*. Chur: Harwood Academic Publishers.

Kent, G. (1996) Shared understandings for informed consent: the relevance of psychological research on provision of information, *Social Science and Medicine*, 43: 1517–23.

Kiebert, G.M., Stiggelbout, A.M., Kieviet, J. et al. (1994) Choices in oncology; factors that influence patients' treatment preference, *Quality of Life Research*, 3: 175–82.

Kimsma, G.K. (1993) Informed consent, in R.J.M. Dillmann, E. van Leeuwen and G.K. Kimsma (eds) *Ethiek in de medische praktijk*. Utrecht: Bunge, pp. 94–106.

Kirby, M. (1983) Informed consent; what does it mean? *Journal of Medical Ethics*, 9: 69–75.

Kleinman, S. and Copp, M.A. (1993) *Emotions and Fieldwork*, Qualitative Research Methods series, vol. 28. London: Sage Publications.

Kloos, P. (1981) *Culturele Antropologie.* Assen: Van Gorcum.
Kloos, P. (1990) Reality and its representations, in P. Kloos (ed.) *True Fiction; Artistic and Scientific Representations of Reality.* Assen: Van Gorcum, pp. 1–6.
Kompanje, E.J.O. (1998) *Medisch-ethische opvattingen en voorwaarden met betrekking tot informed consent.* Utrecht: KNMG (KNMG-Project 'Informed Consent', mr. IC-1).
Kübler-Ross, E. (1969) *Lessen voor levenden; gesprekken met stervenden.* Bilthoven: Ambo.
Lantos, J. (1993) Informed consent: The whole truth for the patients? *Cancer,* 9: 2811–15.
Leenen, H.J.J. (1995) Invoering WGBO; conceptie, groei en geboorte, *Medisch Contact,* 13: 413–14.
Legemaate, J. (1994) *Recht en realiteit.* Houten: Bohn Stafleu Van Loghum.
Legemaate, J. (1995) *De WGBO; van tekst naar toepassing.* Houten: Bohn Stafleu Van Loghum.
Ley, P. (1988) *Communication with Patients. Improving Communication, Satisfaction and Compliance.* London: Chapman and Hall.
McHugh, P., Lewis, S. and Ford, S. (1995) The efficiency of audiotapes in promoting psychological well-being in cancer patients: a randomised, controlled trial, *British Journal of Cancer,* 71: 388–92.
McIntosh, J. (1974) Processes of communication. Information seeking and control associated with cancer: a selective review of literature, *Social Science and Medicine,* 8: 167–87.
McMahan, E., Hoffmann, K. and McGee, G. (1994) Physician-nurse relationships in clinical settings: a review and critique of the literature, 1966–1992, *Medical Care Review,* 51: 83–112.
Maguire, P. and Faulkner, A. (1988a) Communication with cancer patients: 1 Handling bad news and difficult questions, *British Medical Journal,* 297: 907–9.
Maguire, P. and Faulkner, A. (1988b) Communication with cancer patients: 2 Handling uncertainty, collusion, and denial, *British Medical Journal,* 297: 972–4.
Maguire, P. and Faulkner, A. (1988c) Improve the counseling skills of doctors and nurses in cancer care, *British Medical Journal,* 297: 847–9.
Manschot, H. (1994) Kwetsbare autonomie. Over afhankelijkheid en onafhankelijkheid in de ethiek van de zorg, in H. Manschot and M. Verkerk (red.) *Ethiek van de zorg; een discussie.* Amsterdam: Boom, pp. 97–119.
Manschot, H. (1997) Zorg: een blinde vlek in de moderne filosofie, in M. Verkerk (red.) *Denken over zorg; concepten en praktijken.* Utrecht: Elsevier/De Tijdstroom, pp. 49–59.
Mark, J. and Spiro, H. (1990) Informed consent for colonscopy, *Archives of Internal Medicine,* 150: 777–80.
Marshal, V.W. (1980) *Last Chapters: A Sociology of Ageing and Dying.* Monterey, CA: Brooks Cole.
Mays, N. and Pope, C. (1995) Rigour and qualitative research, *British Medical Journal,* 311: 182–4.
Mays, N. and Pope, C. (eds) (1996) *Qualitative Research in Health Care.* London: BMJ Books.

Mol, A. (1997a) Klant, burger, ziek. Het goede in drie talen, in M. Verkerk (red.) *Denken over zorg; concepten en praktijken.* Utrecht: Elsevier/De Tijdstroom, pp. 139–51.

Mol, A. (1997b) *Wat is kiezen?* (oratie).

Nash, A. (1992) Patterns and trends in referrals to a palliative nursing service, *Journal of Advanced Nursing*, 17: 432–40.

Nash, A. (1993) Reasons for referral to a palliative nursing, *Journal of Advanced Nursing*, 18: 7070–13.

Nederlandse kankerbestrijding (1999) *Zorg.* Amsterdam: KWF/NKB.

Novack, D.H., Plumer, R. and Smith, R.L. (1979) Changes in physicians attitude telling the cancer patient, *The Journal of the American Association*, 241(9): 897–900.

Nuland, S.B. (1995) *How We Die: Reflections on Life's Final Chapter.* New York: Vintage Books.

Oakley, A. (1986) Interviewing women: a contradiction in terms? in A. Oakley (ed.) *Telling the Truth about Jerusalem; A Collection of Essays and Poems.* New York: Basil Blackwell, pp. 231–53.

Oken, D. (1961) What to tell cancer patients: a study of medical attitudes, *Journal of the American Medical Association*, 175(13): 1120–8.

Ong, L.M.L., de Haes, J.C.J.M. Hoos, A.M. and Lammes, F.B. (1995) Doctor-patient communication: a review of the literature, *Social Science and Medicine*, 40: 903–18.

Pool, R. (1989) *There must have been something . . . : interpretations of illness and misfortune in a Cameroon Village*, proefschrift, Universiteit van Amsterdam.

Pool, R. (1998) Euthanasie: de stijl van de dokter, in J. Legemaate and R.J.M. Dillmann (red.) *Levensbeëindigend handelen door een arts: tussen norm en praktijk.* Houten: Bohn Stafleu Van Loghum.

Pool, R. (2000) *Negotiating A Good Death: Euthanasia in the Netherlands.* New York: The Haworth Press.

Porter, S. (1991) A participant observation study of power relations between nurses and doctors in a general hospital, *Journal of Advanced Nursing*, 16: 728–35.

Postmus, P.T. (1993) Nieuwvormingen van luchtwegen, longen, mediastinum en pleura, in H.J. Sluyter, M. de Medts, J.H. Dijkman and C. Hilvering (red.) *Longziekten.* Assen/Maastricht: Van Gorcum, pp. 267–303.

Rampen, F.H.J. and van Dam, F.S.A.M. (1987) Informatie aan kankerpatiënten; een onderzoek bij 140 melanoompatiënten, *Medisch Contact*, 16: 507–8.

Redelmeier, D.A., Rozin, P. and Kahneman, D. (1993) Understanding patients decisions; cognitive and emotional perspectives, *Journal of the American Medical Association*, 270: 72–6.

Regt, H.B., de Haan, R.J. and de Haes, J.C.J.M. (1998) *Uitvoering van de informed consent-vereiste; een kwestie van communicatie.* Utrecht: KNMG (KNMG-Project 'Informed Consent', nr. IC-4).

Reinders, H. (1994) De grenzen van het rechtendiscours, in H. Manschot and M. Verkerk (eds) *Ethiek van de zorg; een discussie.* Amsterdam: Boom, pp. 74–97.

Richards, M., Ramirez, A., Degner, L., Fallowfield, L., Maher, L. and Neuberger, J. (1995) Offering choice of treatment to patients with cancer. A review based upon a symposium held at the 10th annual conference of the British Psychosocial Oncology group, *European Journal of Cancer*, 31A: 112–16.

Roscam Abbing, H.D.C. (1993) Het recht op informatie in de medische praktijk, *Nederlands Tijdschrift voor Geneeskunde*, 37: 1861–3.

Roscam Abbing, H.D.C. (1995) Het recht op informatie en het toestemmingsvereiste, in J. Legemaate (red.) *De WGBO: van tekst naar toepassing*. Houten: Bohn Stafleu Van Loghum.

Scholte, B. (1986) The literary turn in contemporary anthropology, *Sociologisch Tijdschrift*, 13/3: 518–38.

Senett, R. (2001) *De Flexibele Mens: Psychogram van de Moderne Samenleving*. Amsterdam: Rainbow.

Sevenhuijsen, S. (1996) *Oordelen met zorg; feministische beschouwingen over recht, moraal en politiek*. Amsterdam/Meppel: Boom.

Shaffir, W.B., Stebbins, R.A. and Turowetz, A. (1980) *Fieldwork Experience: Qualitative Approaches to Social Research*. New York: St. Martin's Press.

Sharma, U. (1996) Using complementary therapies: a challenge to orthodox medicine?, in S.J. Williams and M. Calnan (eds) *Modern Medicine; Lay Perspectives and Experiences*. London: University College London Press.

Shatz, D. (1990) Randomized trials and the problem of suboptimal care: an overview of the controversy, *Cancer Investigation*, 8: 191–205.

Sheehy, D.P. (1973) Rules for dying: A study of alienation and patient-spouse role expectations during terminal illness, *Dissertion Abstracts International*, 33: 3777.

Silverman, W. (1989) The myth of informed consent: in daily practice and in clinical trials, *Journal of Medical Ethics*, 15: 6–11.

Siminoff, L.A., Fetting, J.H. and Abeloff, M.D. (1989) Doctor-patient communication about breast cancer adjuvant therapy, *Journal of Clinical Oncology*, 9: 1192–200.

Siminoff, L.A. and Fetting, J.H. (1991) Factors affecting treatment decisions for a life-threatening illness: the case of medical treatment of breast cancer, *Social Science of Medicine*, 32: 813–18.

Slevin, M.L., Stubbs, L., Plant, H.J. et al. (1990) Attitudes to chemotherapy; comparing views of patients with cancer with those of doctors, nurses, and general public, *British Medical Journal*, 330: 1458–60.

Smith Bowen, E. (1956) *Return to Laughter*. London: Gollanz.

Solzehenitsyn, A. (1968) *Het kankerpaviljoen, deel 1 en 2*. Baarn: Boekerij.

Stein, L., Watts, D. and Howell, T. (1990) The doctor-nurse game revisited, *New England Journal of Medicine*, 322: 446–9.

Steward, M. (1983) Patient characteristics with related to the doctor-patient interaction, *Family Practice*.

Steward, M.A. (1984) What is a successful doctor-patient interview? A study of interactions and outcomes, *Social Science and Medicine*, 19: 167–75.

Street, R.L. Jr. (1991) Information-giving in medical consultations: the influence of patients' communicative styles and personal characteristics, *Social Science and Medicine*, 32(5): 541–8.

Stüsgen, R.A.J. (1995) Tussen volgzaamheid en autonomie, *Medisch Contact*, 50: 821–3.

Sudnow, D. (1967) *Passing On*. New Jersey: Prentice Hall.

Sulmasy, D., Lehman, D., Levine, D. and Faden, R. (1994) Patients perception of the quality of informed consent for common medical procedures. Special section:

Informed consent in clinical practice, *The Journal of Clinical Ethics*, 5: 189–94, 243–50.

Sutherland, H.J., Llewellyn-Thomas, H.A., Lockwood, G.A., Tritchler, D.L. and Till, J.E. (1989) Cancer patients: their desire for information and participation in treatment decisions, *Journal of the Royal Society of Medicine*, 82: 260–3.

Tannen, D. (1993) *Hoe taal relaties maakt of breekt*. Amsterdam: Prometheus.

Taylor, K.M. (1984) 'Telling bad news': physicians and the disclosure of undesirable information, *Sociology of Health and Illness*, 10: 109–32.

ten Kroode, H.F.J. (1990) *Het verhaal van kankerpatienten: oorzaakstoekenning en betekenisverlening. een onderzoek naar het verband tussen attributies en zelfrespect*, proefschrift, Rijksuniversiteit Utrecht.

ter Borg, M. (1993) *De dood als het einde; een cultuur-sociologisch essay*. Baarn: Ten Have.

The, B.A.M., Koëter, G.H., Timstra, Tj. and Groen, H.J.M. (1996) 'Wij kunnen u wel behandelen': communicatie met patiënten met een kleincellig, bronchuscarcinoom (klinische les), *Nederlands Tijdschrift voor Geneeskunde*, 140(41): 2021–3.

The, B.A.M. (1997a) *'Vanavond om 8 uur . . .', verpleegkundige dilemma's bij euthanasie en andere beslissingen rond het levenseinde*. Houten: Bohn Stafleu Van Loghum.

The, B.A.M. (1997b) Op zoek naar de juiste balans tussen distantie en betrokkenheid; veldwerkervaringen van een cultureel antropologe in een ziekenhuis, in Goethals, A., Hak, T. and ten Have, P. (ed.) *Kwalitatieve medische sociologie*. Amsterdam: SISWO, pp. 139–57.

The, B.A.M. (1998) Verpleegkundige dilemma's bij euthanasie en andere beslissingen rondom het levenseinde, in J. Legemaate and R.J.M. Dillmann (red.) *Levensbeëindigend handelen door een arts: tussen norm en praktijk*. Houten: Bohn Stafleu Van Loghum.

The, B.A.M., Hak, A., Koëter, G.H. and van der Wal, G. (2001) Collusion in doctor-patient communication about imminent death: an ethnographic study, *British Medical Journal*, 321: 1376–81.

Thomas, J. (1993) *Doing Critical Ethnography*. Qualitative Research Methods series, vol. 26. London: Sage Publications.

Tijmstra, Tj. (1987) Het imperatieve karakter van medische technologie en de betekenis van 'geanticipeerde beslissingsspijt', *Nederlands Tijdschrift voor Geneeskunde*, 131: 1128–31.

van Busschbach, J.T. (1986) *Patiëntenvoorlichting gemeten. Ontwikkeling en toepassing van een observatie-instrument*. Utrecht: NIVEL.

van den e.a. Burg, W. (1994) The care of a good caregiver: legal end ethical reflections on the good healthcare professional, *Cambridge Quarterly of Healthcare Ethics*, 3: 38–48.

van Dantzig, A. (1993) Medische zorg alleen maakt niet gelukkig!, in H.J. de Ruyter and M.J. Mineur (eds) *De achterkant van de medische zorg; over de keerzijde van de medisch-technische medaille*. Groningen: AZG.

van Wijmen, F.C.B. (1995) Vertrouwen en verantwoorde zorg; bij de inwerkingtreding van de WGBO, *Medisch Contact*, 13: 411–12.

van der Zouwe, N. (1994) *Alternatieve kankertherapieën* (proefschrift).

van Uden, M.M.A. and van Dam, F.S.A.M. (1986) Informed consent bij klinisch kankeronderzoek; psychologische aspecten, *Nederlands Tijdschrift voor Geneeskunde*, 130(46): 2078–82.

Varekamp, I., Koedoot, C.G., Bakker, P.J.M., de Graeff, A. and de Haes, J.C.J.M. (1997) Gezamenlijk beslissen, hoezo? (klinische les), *Nederlands Tijdschrift voor Geneeskunde*, 141: 1897–1900.

Verbeek-Heida, P. (1998) 'De nieuwe patiënt op weg naar autonomie' (recentie proefschrift R. Stüsgen), Kwalon. *Tijschrift voor kwalitatief onderzoek in Nederland*, 3(8): 46–50.

Verhaak, P.F.M., Andela, M. and Kerstens, J.J. (1986) Bejegening en informatieverstrekking door huisarts en specialist. De visie van de patiënt, *Medisch Contact*, 26: 864–6.

Verheggen, F. (1996) *Myth and reality of informed consent and the patient's choice to participate in clinical trials*. Proefschrift. Maastricht: UPM.

Verkerk, M. (1994) Zorg of contract: een andere ethiek, in H. Manschot and M. Verker (red.) *Ethiek van de zorg; een discussie*. Amsterdam: Boom, pp. 53–74.

Verkerk, M. (1996) *Mijnheer, heb ik met u een zorgrelatie? Over ethiek, over zorg en over een ethiek van de zorg*. (oratie).

Verkerk, M. (1997) Een ethiek van kwetsbaarheid; over verzwegen premisse, in M. Verkerk (red.) *Denken over zorg; concepten en praktijken*. Utrecht: Elsevier/De Tijdstroom, pp. 87–103.

Verkerk, M. (2000) Een pleidooi voor zorg voor zichzelf. Trouw juli.

Vroegop, P. and Burghouts, J.T.M. (1989) Levensverlenging door cytostatica: de moeite waard? Een vragenlijstonderzoek bij nabestaanden, *Nederlands Tijdschrift voor Geneeskunde*, 133: 2173–7.

Wagener, D.J.Th. (1987) De ongeneeslijk zieke patiënt door de ogen van een clinicus, *Nederlands Tijdschrift voor Geneeskunde*, 131: 1004–8.

Wagener, D.J.Th. (1996) *Slecht nieuws; een handreiking bij de gespreksvoering*. Utrecht: Bunge.

Wagener, J.J. and Taylor, S.E. (1986) What else could I have done? Patients' responses to failed treatment decisions, *Health Psychology*, 5: 481–96.

Waitzkin, H. (1985) Information giving in medical care, *Journal of Health and Social Behavior*, 26: 81–101.

Wear, S. (1993) *Informed Consent: Patient Autonomy and Physician Benefits within Clinical Medicine*. Dordrecht: Kluwer.

Williams, R. (1989) Awareness and control of dying; some paradoxical trends in public opinion, *Sociology of Health and Illness*, 11: 201–12.

Wolffers, I. (1995) Kwalitatieve benaderingen in het medisch onderzoek, *Nederlands Tijdschrift voor Geneeskunde*, 139: 2580–3.

Zussman, R. (1992) *Intensive Care: Medical Ethics and the Medical Profession*. Chicago, IL: The University of Chicago Press.

Zuuren, F.J. (1995) Kwalitatief onderzoek; het belang van een kwalitatieve benadering bij onderzoek in de sociale gezondheidszorg, *Tijdschrift voor Sociale Gezondheidszorg*, 7: 315–21.

Index

illness trajectory (first phase)
  doctors' perspectives, 3, 29–39
  nurses' perspectives, 3, 39–43
  patients' perspectives, 3, 9–28
illness trajectory (second phase)
  optimism about recovery, 66–79
  patient uncertainty/anxiety, 80–8
  rescue therapy (very sick patient),
    57–65
  rising curve (developing calm),
    47–56
illness trajectory (third phase)
  declining optimism, 109–29
  patient has more chemotherapy,
    91–108
  patient stops chemotherapy, 130–8
impression management, 79
infection, 118–20, 134
information
  bad news, see bad news interview
  long-term perspective, 194–7,
    199–201, 207–8, 221, 222, 224
  pattern of provision, 122–4, 194
  perspective, 4, 219
  provision (styles), 148–50
  public/hidden, 197–200, 207–8, 221
  short-term perspective, 194–9, 201,
    207–8, 221, 222
informed consent, 2, 23, 33, 35–6,
  189, 214–20
intellectual patients, 33, 38–9, 72–3,
  100, 208–9, 211
intensive care (IC) ward, 74, 226
invisible information, 197–200
involuntary play acting (nurses), 77–8
irradiated water, 52, 82, 87
Iwashyna, T.J., 223

jargon, 69–70
Jaspers, Dr, 24
joint consultations, 74
Jomande (faith healer), 53
Jonker, Nanet (nurse), 27
'judging with care', 219
junior doctors, 106, 117, 148, 228

Kassies, Mrs (patient), 38
Katz Rothman, B., 235

Kellehear, A., 12, 21, 78, 79, 158,
  172n, 183, 198, 205n, 207
Kompanje, E.J.O., 210, 211
Kooiman, Dr Menno, 15, 16, 18–20,
  21, 83, 93, 114, 124
Kornelisse, Mirjam (nurse), 144, 150
Korte, Dr Jacob, 61
Koster, Mr (patient), 50, 66–7, 230
  anxiety and reflection, 85–6, 87
  declining optimism, 109–11, 120, 126
  parting, 177–9, 185
Kramer, Lotte (nurse), 173, 175
Kübler-Ross, E., 22, 172n
Kuipers, Mira (nurse), 57, 58, 59, 60,
  62, 64

language/language use, 4, 65, 69–71
latent realization of death, 207–9
Law on Medical-Scientific Research with
  Human Subjects, 214, 217, 218
lecture (patient's role), 95, 98–9, 103
Leenen, H.J.J., 2
Legemaate, J., 2, 215–16
legislation, 2, 214, 215–17, 218
leucocytes, 143
leukopenic ascites, 58, 60, 141
Ley, P., 69n
Liem, Dr Guido, 1, 2, 196n, 230,
  232–3
  bad news interview, 10–12, 14,
    20–1, 24–7, 29–35, 38, 40
  lecture, 95, 98–9, 103
  response to parting, 143, 146–7,
    149–50, 152–7, 159–60, 165,
    175, 177–82
  response to patients in therapy,
    50–1, 55, 57, 70, 74
  response to recurrences, 92–9, 101,
    103–5, 108–13, 116–19, 121–4,
    130–1, 133–7
life experience/style, 22–3, 184, 185
limited disease, 30
locums, 148
Loman, Dr Mariane, 143
long-term perspective, 194–7,
  199–201, 207–8, 221, 222, 224
loyalty (toward doctor), 40, 42–3,
  99–100

AN INTIMATE DEATH
SUPPORTING BEREAVED PARENTS AND SIBLINGS

Gordon Riches and Pam Dawson

- What impact does a child's death have on family relationships?
- How might differences in the way mothers and fathers deal with bereavement contribute to increased marital tension?
- Why are bereaved siblings so deeply affected by the way their parents grieve?

An Intimate Loneliness explores how family members attempt to come to terms with the death of an offspring or brother or sister. Drawing on relevant research and the authors' own experience of working with bereaved parents and siblings, this book examines the importance of social relationships in helping them adjust to their bereavement. The chances of making sense of this most distressing loss are influenced by the resilience of the family's surviving relationships, by the availability of wider support networks and by the cultural resources that inform each's perception of death. This book considers the impact of bereavement on self and family identity. In particular, it examines the role of shared remembering in transforming survivors' relationships with the deceased, and in helping rebuild their own identity with a significantly changed family structure. Problems considered include: the failure of intimate relationships, cultural and gender expectations, the 'invisibility' of fathers' and siblings' grief, sudden and 'difficult' deaths, lack of information, and the sense of isolation felt by some family members.

This book will be of value to students on courses in counselling, health care, psychology, social policy, pastoral care and education. It will appeal to sociology students with an interest in death, dying and mortality. It is also aimed at professionally qualified counselling, health and social service workers, informed voluntary group members, the clergy, teachers and others involved with pastoral care.

Contents
Introduction: an intimate loneliness – Order out of chaos: personal, social and cultural resources for making sense of loss – A bleak and lonely landscape: problems of adjustment for bereaved parents – What about me? Problems of adjustment for bereaved siblings – Connnections and disconnections: ways family members deal with lost relationships – Difficult death and problems of adjustment – Things that help: supporting bereaved parents and brothers and sisters – Conclusion: professional support in a post-modern world – Appendix: Shoe-strings and bricolage: some notes on the background research project – References – Index.

240pp   0 335 19972 0 (Paperback)   0 335 19973 9 (Hardback)

ON BEREAVEMENT
THE CULTURE OF GRIEF

Tony Walter

Insightful and refreshing.
Professor Dennis Klass, Webster University, St Louis, USA

A tour de force.
Dr Colin Murray Parkes, OBE, MD, FRCPsych,
President of CRUSE

Some societies and some individuals find a place for their dead, others leave them behind. In recent years, researchers, professionals and bereaved people themselves have struggled with this. Should the band with the dead be continued or broken? What is clear is that the grieving individual is not left in a social vacuum but has to struggle with expectations from self, family, friends, professionals and academic theorists.

This ground-breaking book looks at the social position of the bereaved. They find themselves caught between the living and the dead, sometimes searching for guidelines in a de-ritualized society that has few to offer, sometimes finding their grief inappropriately pathologized and policed. At its best, bereavement care offers reassurance, validation and freedom to talk where the client has previously encountered judgmentalism.

In this unique book, Tony Walter applies sociological insights to one of the most personal of human situations. *On Bereavement* is aimed at students on medical, nursing, counselling and social work courses that include bereavement as a topic. It will also appeal to sociology students with an interest in death, dying and mortality.

Contents
Introduction – Part I: Living with the dead – Other places, other times – War, peace and the dead: twentieth-century ppular culture – Private bonds – Public bonds: the dead in everyday conversation – The last chapter –Theories – Part II: Policing grief – Guidelines for grief: historical background – Popular guidelines: the English case – Expert guidelines: clinical lore – Vive la différence? The politics of gender – Bereavement care – Conclusion: integration, regulation and postmodernism – References – Index.

256pp   0 335 20080 X (Paperback)   0 335 20081 8 (Hardback)

REFLECTIONS ON PALLIATIVE CARE

David Clark and Jane E. Seymour

Palliative care seems set to continue its rapid development into the early years of the twenty-first century. From its origins in the modern hospice movement, the new multidisciplinary specialty of palliative care has expanded into a variety of settings. Palliative care services are now being provided in the home, in hospital and in nursing homes. There are moves to extend palliative care beyond its traditional constituency of people with cancer. Efforts are being made to provide a wide range of palliative therapies to patients at an early stage of their disease progression. The evidence-base of palliative care is growing, with more research, evaluation and audit, along with specialist programmes of education. Palliative care appears to be coming of age.

On the other hand numbers of challenges still exist. Much service development has been unplanned and unregulated. Palliative care providers must continue to adapt to changing patterns of commissioning and funding services. The voluntary hospice movement may feel its values threatened by a new professionalism and policies which require its greater integration within mainstream services. There are concerns about the re-medicalization of palliative care, about how an evidence-based approach to practice can be developed, and about the extent to which its methods are transferring across diseases and settings.

Beyond these preoccupations lie wider societal issues about the organization of death and dying in late modern culture. To what extent have notions of death as a contemporary taboo been superseded? How can we characterize the nature of suffering? What factors are involved in the debate surrounding end of life care ethics and euthanasia?

David Clark and Jane Seymour, drawing on a wide range of sources, as well as their own empirical studies, offer a set of reflections on the development of palliative care and its place within a wider social context. Their book will be essential reading to any practitioner, policy maker, teacher or student involved in palliative care or concerned about death, dying and life-limiting illness.

Contents
Introduction – Part I: Death in society – The social meaning of death and suffering – Ageing, dying and grieving – The ethics of dying – Part II: The philosophy and practice of palliative care – History and development – Definitions, components, meanings – Routinization and medicalization – Part III: Policy issues – Policy development and palliative care – The delivery of palliative care services – Part IV: Conclusion – The future for palliative care – References – Index.

224pp   0 335 19454 0 (Paperback)   0 335 19455 9 (Hardback)